Contemporary Diabetes

Series Editor: Aristidis Veves

For further volumes:
http://www.springer.com/series/7679

Samy I. McFarlane • George L. Bakris
Editors

Diabetes and Hypertension

Evaluation and Management

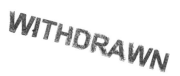

☼ Humana Press

Editors
Samy I. McFarlane, MD, MPH, MBA
Division of Endocrinology, Diabetes and
Hypertension, Department of Medicine
SUNY-Downstate and Kings County
Hospital
Brooklyn, NY, USA

George L. Bakris, MD
ASH Comprehensive Hypertension Center
Department of Medicine
University of Chicago Medical Center
Chicago, IL, USA

ISBN 978-1-60327-356-5   ISBN 978-1-60327-357-2 (eBook)
DOI 10.1007/978-1-60327-357-2
Springer New York Heidelberg Dordrecht London

Library of Congress Control Number: 2012948136

Printed on acid-free paper

Humana Press is a brand of Springer
Springer is part of Springer Science+Business Media (www.springer.com)

Preface

Diabetes and hypertension have evolved as two of the modern day epidemics affecting millions of people around the globe. These two common comorbidities lead to substantial increase in cardiovascular disease, the major cause of morbidity and mortality of adults around the world.

Physicians and other health care providers are increasingly encountering patients with diabetes and hypertension in their practice. This book consists of 14 chapters written by top authorities in their respective fields. Topics covered range from basic concepts in evaluation and management of diabetes and hypertension such as dietary interventions to evaluation and management of secondary hypertension in clinical practice. Other chapters focus on high cardiovascular risk populations such as those with coronary heart disease, chronic kidney disease, and minority patients.

Finally, evolving concepts and new developments in the field are presented in other chapters such as prevention of type 2 diabetes and the epidemic of sleep apnea and its implication for diabetes and hypertension evaluation and management.

We hope that this book will provide the busy practitioner with cutting-edge knowledge in the field as well as practical information that would translate into better care provided to such high risk population of diabetics and hypertensive patients.

Brooklyn, NY, USA   Samy I. McFarlane, MD, MPH, MBA
Chicago, IL, USA   George L. Bakris, MD

Contents

Contributors

Monsur Adedayo Department of Medicine, Sleep Disorder and Disparity Centers, SUNY Downstate Medical Center, Brooklyn, NY, USA

George L. Bakris, M.D. Department of Medicine, ASH Comprehensive Hypertension Center, University of Chicago Medical Center, Chicago, IL, USA

Joshua Botdorf Department of Internal Medicine, University of Missouri-Columbia School of Medicine, Columbia, MO, USA

Walter A. Brzezinski Division of General Internal Medicine, Department of Medicine, Medical University of South Carolina, Charleston, SC, USA

Jaya P. Buddineni, M.D. Department of General Internal Medicine, University of Missouri-Columbia School of Medicine, Columbia, MO, USA

Kunal Chaudhary, M.D. Division of Nephrology and Hypertension, Harry S. Truman VA Medical Center, Columbia, MO, USA

Department of Internal Medicine, University of Missouri-Columbia School of Medicine, Columbia, MO, USA

Lorena Drago, M.S., R.D., C.D.N., C.D.E. Diabetes Education Program, Lincoln Medical and Mental Health Center, New York, NY, USA

Brent M. Egan, M.D. Division of General Internal Medicine, Department of Medicine, Medical University of South Carolina, Charleston, SC, USA

Mariana Garcia-Touza Division of Endocrinology, Diabetes and Metabolism, Department of Internal Medicine, University of Missouri-Columbia School of Medicine, Columbia, MO, USA

Haisam Ismail, M.D. Department of Cardiology, Hofstra North Shore-LIJ School of Medicine, North Shore University Hospital, Manhasset, NY, USA

Girardin Jean-Louis, Ph.D. Department of Medicine, Sleep Disorder and Disparity Centers, SUNY-Downstate, Brooklyn, NY, USA

Jocelyne G. Karam, M.D. Division of Endocrinology, Maimonides Medical Center, SUNY-Downstate College of Medicine, Brooklyn, NY, USA

Ivana Lazich, M.D. Department of Medicine, ASH Comprehensive Hypertension Center, University of Chicago, Medical Center, Chicago, IL, USA

Douglas R. Lazzaro, M.D., F.A.C.S., F.A.A.O. Department of Ophthalmology, The Richard C. Troutman, M.D. Distinguished Chair in Ophthalmology and Ophthalmic Microsurgery, SUNY Downstate Medical Center, Brooklyn, NY 11203, USA

UHB, SUNY Downstate Medical Center, Brooklyn, NY 11203, USA

KCHC, HHC, Brooklyn, NY 11203, USA

LICH, SUNY Downstate Medical Center, Brooklyn, NY 11203, USA

Edgar Lerma Section of Nephrology, University of Illinois at Chicago School of Medicine, Chicago, IL, USA

Sidrah Mahmud Department of Medicine, Sleep Disorder and Disparity Centers, SUNY Downstate Medical Center, Brooklyn, NY, USA

Amgad N. Makaryus, M.D. Department of Cardiology, Hofstra North Shore-LIJ School of Medicine, North Shore University Hospital, Manhasset, NY, USA

Samy I. McFarlane, M.D., M.P.H., M.B.A. Division of Endocrinology, Diabetes and Hypertension, Department of Medicine, SUNY-Downstate and Kings County Hospital, Brooklyn, NY, USA

Gbenga Ogedegbe, M.D. Division of General Internal Medicine, Department of Medicine, Center for Healthful Behavior Change, New York University School of Medicine, New York, NY, USA

Oladipupo Olafiranye Division of Cardiology, Department of Medicine, SUNY Downstate Medical Center, Brooklyn, NY, USA

Abhishek Pandey Department of Medicine, Sleep Disorder and Disparity Centers, SUNY Downstate Medical Center, Brooklyn, NY, USA

Mahboob Rahman, M.D., M.S. Division of Nephrology and Hypertension, Case Western Reserve University, Cleveland, OH, USA

Eric Shrier, M.D. Department of Ophthalmology, SUNY Downstate Medical Center, Brooklyn, NY, USA

James R. Sowers, M.D. Division of Endocrinology, Diabetes and Metabolism, Department of Internal Medicine, University of Missouri-Columbia School of Medicine, Columbia, MO, USA

Harry S. Truman Memorial Veterans' Hospital, Columbia, MO, USA

Adam Whaley-Connell Division of Nephrology and Hypertension, Harry S. Truman VA Medical Center, Columbia, MO, USA

Department of Internal Medicine, University of Missouri-Columbia School of Medicine, Columbia, MO, USA

Nathaniel Winer, M.D. Department of Medicine, Division of Endocrinology, SUNY Downstate Medical Center, Brooklyn, NY, USA

Yumin Zhao Division of General Internal Medicine, Department of Medicine, Medical University of South Carolina, Charleston, SC, USA

Ferdinand Zizi Department of Medicine, Sleep Disorder and Disparity Centers, SUNY-Downstate Medical Center, Brooklyn, NY, USA

Chapter 1
Epidemiology of Hypertension in Diabetes

Brent M. Egan, Yumin Zhao, and Walter A. Brzezinski

Prevalent hypertension, defined by average blood pressure (BP) $\geq 140/\geq 90$ mmHg or self-reported treatment, is more common among diabetic patients than the general population [1, 2]. In fact, the prevalence of hypertension among diabetics was reportedly twice that of the general U.S. population of adults in 2005–2008 at 57.3% versus 28.6% [2]. Diabetes approximately doubles risk for cardiovascular disease and concomitant hypertension nearly doubles that risk again [3–7]. As a result, the treatment and control of hypertension in diabetes receive special attention in several professional guideline reports [8–10].

Previous publications addressed the clinical epidemiology of hypertension in patients with diabetes [1, 2, 11, 12]. All reports defined prevalent hypertension as indicated above. Hypertension control among treated diabetics did not change, and if anything tended to decline between 1988–1991 and, 1999–2000 at $<140/<90$ (53.1 vs. 46.9) and $<130/<85$ (28.5 vs. 25.4), although the differences were not statistically significant [11]. Among diabetic hypertensives on treatment, age-adjusted BP control to $<130/<80$ improved from 15.7% in 1999–2000 to 37.5% in 2003–2004 [12].

In 1999–2000, BP control to $<140/<90$ was documented in 53.1% of all treated hypertensives and 46.9% among all treated hypertensive diabetics [11]. In contrast, by 2005–2008, BP control to $<140/<90$ among all hypertensives was higher among those with diabetes than those without diabetes (56.9% vs. 41.7%, $p < 0.05$) [2]. These reports cannot be directly compared as the methodologies, while acceptable, were not standardized.

B.M. Egan, M.D. (✉) • Y. Zhao • W.A. Brzezinski
Division of General Internal Medicine, Department of Medicine, Medical University
of South Carolina, 135 Rutledge Avenue, RT1230, Charleston, SC 29425, USA
e-mail: eganbm@musc.edu

S.I. McFarlane and G.L. Bakris (eds.), *Diabetes and Hypertension: Evaluation and Management*, Contemporary Diabetes, DOI 10.1007/978-1-60327-357-2_1,
© Springer Science+Business Media New York 2012

Hypertension control is critically important for ameliorating vascular risk among diabetic hypertensives [8–10]. Time trends in the clinical epidemiology of hypertension in diabetics may be useful in informing and guiding healthcare policy, professional guidelines, and quality improvement programs to optimize health outcomes. This report attempts to address a gap in the clinical epidemiology of hypertension among patients with diabetes using the same methods reported previously [13].

Methods

As described previously [13], NHANES 1988–1994 and 1999–2008 were conducted by the Centers for Disease Control and Prevention National Center for Health Statistics (NCHS). NHANES participants were identified using stratified, multistage probability sampling of the noninstitutionalized US population. All participating adults provided written consent approved by the NCHS Institutional/Ethics Review Board.

Definitions

Race/ethnicity was determined by self-report as non-Hispanic white (white), non-Hispanic black (black), and Hispanic ethnicity, and other race as described.

Blood pressure (BP) measurement methods were consistent across the NHANES included in this report [13]. In brief, BP was measured by trained physicians using a mercury sphygmomanometer and appropriately sized arm cuff on subjects after 5 min seated rest. Individuals without recorded BP were excluded. In calculating mean systolic and diastolic BP for individuals, the first BP value was used if only one measurement was obtained. The second BP was used if two readings were taken; the second and third values were averaged when available. More than 90% of participants had two or more measurements of BP in all NHANES periods included in this report. As described, excluding the first BP when ≥2 measurements are taken results in a lower BP value [13].

Hypertension was defined as mean systolic BP ≥140 and/or mean diastolic BP ≥90 mmHg and/or a positive response to the question "Are you currently taking medication to lower your BP?" [11–13] *Hypertension awareness* was determined by hypertensive patients responding affirmatively to the question, "Have you ever been told by a doctor or other healthcare professional that you had hypertension, also called high BP?" [11–13] Hypertension treatment was established by participants responding "Yes" to the question, "Because of your hypertension/high BP are you now taking prescribed medicine?" [11–13]

Control of hypertension was defined as BP <140/<90 mmHg across all survey periods, although the BP goals for high-risk subgroups including diabetics were lower for 1999–2008. [11–13]. Recent evidence does not clearly support a goal systolic BP lower than the long established level of <140 for patients with diabetes [14]. For these reasons and to facilitate comparisons across studies, this report focuses mainly on goal BP <140/<90.

Diabetes mellitus was defined by an affirmative response to the questions, "Have you ever been told by a doctor that you have diabetes?," and/or "Are you now taking insulin?," and/or "Are you now taking diabetes pills to lower your blood sugar?" [11–13] The definition did not include "undiagnosed diabetes" based on fasting glucose only.

Antihypertensive medications. Participants were asked if they had taken any prescription medications in the past month. During the household surveys in 1999–2004 and 2005–2008, participants were requested to provide prescription containers and 88.8% and 88.3%, respectively, did so. Each medication identified from medications provided or described was recorded and matched to a prescription drug database. Each medication identified was assigned its generic equivalent. Antihypertensive medications were classified to a single category according to the Seventh Report of the Joint National Committee on Hypertension with addition of proprietary medications not marketed when the document was published [15]. Single-pill combinations were separated into their generic components. Each medication was classified to only one category. The sum of BP medication categories defined the number of antihypertensive medications taken.

Data Analysis

The NHANES Analytic and Reporting Guidelines were followed [16, 17]. SAS callable SUDAAN version 9.0.1 (Cary, NC) was used to account for the complex NHANES sampling design. Standard errors were estimated using Taylor series linearization. All NHANES periods were age adjusted to the U.S. 2000 census data [13, 14].

To test for significant differences in variables between/among groups within each survey, the Chi-Square test in the CROSSTAB procedure was used for categorical variables; WALD F test in the REGRESS was used for continuous variables. When more than two groups were compared within an NHANES survey period, analysis was limited to assessing differences across the groups and not between pairs. Pair-wise comparisons between the three NHANES periods were conducted using *t*-tests of weighted means [1] between pairs of the three groups. The effects of time were not assessed before pair-wise comparisons as SUDAAN would not allow this function when only three time periods were analyzed. Since multiple statistical comparisons were performed within and between the three NHANES time periods, two-sided *p*-values <0.01 were accepted as statistically significant.

Results

Patients with diabetes and hypertension (Table 1.1). Diabetic hypertensives had a mean age of 62.5–63.7 years across surveys (Table 1.1). Mean BP among all diabetic hypertensives declined from 145.2/74.7 in 1988–1994 to 136.5/69.7 mmHg. The proportion of patients with normal BP <120/<80 and "Stage 1" pre-hypertension (120–129/80–84) rose, whereas the percentage with Stage 2 hypertension fell over time. Mean body mass index increased over the survey periods, while the proportion of subjects who were lean and overweight declined and the proportion that were obese increased.

Controlled and uncontrolled diabetic hypertensives (Table 1.2). With hypertension control defined as a BP <140/<90 mmHg, the proportion of controlled patients rose from 35.5% in 1988–1994 to 54.6% in 2005–2008. Systolic BP did not change significantly over time in either controlled or uncontrolled patients, whereas

Table 1.1 Characteristics of patients with diabetes and hypertension in three NHANES periods

	NHANES time period		
	1988–1994 $n=783$	1999–2004 $n=886$	2005–2008 $n=842$
Mean age (years)	63.7 (62.3, 65.1)	62.6 (61.3, 63.9)	62.5 (60.9, 64.0)
Sex (%)			
Men	36.6 (31.8, 41.6)*	45.0 (41.2, 48.8)	43.7 (38.6, 49.0)
Women	63.4 (58.4, 68.2)	55.0 (51.2, 58.8)	56.3 (51.0, 61.4)
Race/ethnicity (%)			
White	72.3 (67.6, 76.5)	65.3 (58.7, 71.4)	65.0 (57.5, 71.8)
Black	17.9 (14.5, 21.9)	18.1 (13.8, 23.2)	20.1 (14.8, 26.6)
Hispanic	5.1 (4.3, 6.2)*	12.6 (8.1, 19.3)	10.6 (7.2, 15.3)*
Others	4.7 (2.7, 8.1)	4.0 (2.3, 6.9)	4.4 (2.6, 7.2)
Mean BP (mmHg)			
Systolic	145.2 (142.2, 148.2)**	139.0 (137.3, 140.8)	136.5 (134.5, 138.6)**
Diastolic	74.7 (73.0, 76.4)**	70.2 (68.6, 71.7)	69.7 (68.0, 71.3)**
BP (mmHg) (%)			
<120/80	10.7 (7.1, 15.8)	16.8 (13.8, 20.2)	20.8 (16.7, 25.6)**
120–129/80–84	9.6 (6.8, 13.4)	13.4 (10.4, 17.1)	16.5 (13.8, 19.8)**
130–139/85–89	15.2 (11.6, 19.5)	18.6 (16.2, 21.3)	17.3 (14.1, 21)
120–139/80–89	24.8 (20.6, 29.5)*	32.0 (28.5, 35.8)	33.8 (30.1, 37.8)**
140–159/90–99	41.0 (35.1, 47.1)	33 (29.4, 36.8)	30.9 (26.5, 35.6)*
≥160/≥100	23.5 (19.6, 28.0)	18.2 (15, 21.8)	14.5 (11.4, 18.2)*
Mean BMI (kg/m^2)	31.3 (30.6, 32.0)	32.6 (31.8, 33.3)	33.1 (32.4, 33.7)**
BMI (%)			
<25	16.3 (13.2, 19.9)	12.4 (9.4, 16.1)	13.0 (10.7, 15.6)
25.0–29.9	33.3 (29.1, 37.7)	28.5 (24.7, 32.7)	25.9 (22.2, 30.1)*
≥30	50.4 (45.5, 55.4)*	59.1 (54.1, 63.9)	61.1 (56.9, 65.1)**

BP blood pressure, *BMI* body mass index
*$p<0.01$, **$p<0.001$. Symbols in column 1 (1988–1994) denote difference versus column 2 (1999–2004). Symbols in column 3 (2005–2008) indicate differences versus column 1. No significant differences were observed for any variable between columns 2 and 3

Table 1.2 Characteristics of controlled and uncontrolled patients with diabetes and hypertension in three NHANES time periods

	1988–1994		1999–2004		2005–2008	
	Controlled	Uncontrolled	Controlled	Uncontrolled	Controlled	Uncontrolled
Number (%) (95% CI)	231	552	399	487	460	382
Mean age (years)	35.5 (29.7–41.7)	64.5 (58.3, 70.3)	48.8 (44.7, 52.9)	51.2 (47.1, 55.3)	54.6 (50, 59.2)	45.4 (40.8, 50.0)
Sex (%)						
Men	35.5 (27.6–44.3)*	37.1 (31, 43.7)	49.0 (41.5, 56.5)	41.2 (36.6, 46)	45.2 (38.0, 52.6)	41.9 (36.2, 47.9)
Women	64.5 (55.7–72.4)	62.9 (56.3, 69)	51.0 (43.5, 58.5)	58.8 (54, 63.4)	54.8 (47.4, 62)	58.1 (52.1, 63.8)
Race/ethnicity (%)						
White	77.1 (70.1–82.8)	69.6 (63.7, 75.0)	67.6 (59.1, 75.1)	63.1 (55.6, 70.1)	65.7 (57.7, 72.9)	64.1 (55.5, 71.8)
Black	16.1 (11.8–21.7)	18.9 (14.8, 23.7)	17.0 (12.8, 22.3)	19.0 (13.7, 25.8)	20.0 (14.8, 26.5)	20.2 (14, 28.2)
Hispanic	3.8 (2.3–6.0)*	5.9 (4.8, 7.3)	12.3 (7.2, 20.2)	13 (7.6, 21.1)	9.6 (6.5, 13.9)*	11.8 (7.6, 17.8)
Others	3.1 (0.9–9.7)	5.6 (2.5, 12)	3.0 (1.5, 6.1)	4.9 (2.5, 9.3)	4.7 (2.2, 9.7)	4.0 (2.1, 7.5)
Mean BP (mmHg)						
Systolic	123.4 (121.5–125.3)	157.2§ (154.2, 160.3)	122.8 (121.2, 124.4)	154.5§ (152.8, 156.2)	121.2 (119.6, 122.8)	155.0§ (152.8, 157.1)
Diastolic	70.6 (68.5, 72.8)*	77.0 (75.0, 79.0)§	66.4 (64.6, 68.2)	73.7 (71.5, 75.9)‡§	65.9 (64.4, 67.5)‡	74.1 (71.7, 76.6)§
BP (mmHg) (%)						
<120/80	30.2 (21.7, 40.3)	0§	34.4 (29, 40.1)	0§	38.1 (31.8, 44.8)	0§
120–129/80–84	27.1 (18.7, 37.5)	0	27.5 (22, 33.7)	0	30.3 (24.9, 36.3)	0
130–139/85–89	42.7 (34.7, 51.2)	0	38.2 (33, 43.7)	0	31.6 (26.1, 37.8)	0
120–139/80–89	69.8 (59.7, 78.3)	0	65.6 (59.9, 71)	0	61.9 (55.2, 68.2)	0
140–159/90–99	0	63.5 (57.1, 69.5)	0	64.5 (58.6, 69.9)	0	68.1 (60.9, 74.5)
≥160/100	0	36.5 (30.5, 42.9)	0	35.5 (30.1, 41.4)	0	31.9 (25.5, 39.1)
Mean BMI (kg/m²)	32.9 (31.6, 34.3)	30.5 (29.7, 31.2)‡	33.2 (32.3, 34.1)	31.9 (30.9, 32.9)	33.9 (33.1, 34.7)	32.1 (30.7, 33.5)
BMI (%)						
<25	10.8 (6.4, 17.6)	19.4 (15.8, 23.5)	9.0 (5.2, 15.3)	15.5 (10.5, 22.3)‡	9.7 (7, 13.3)	16.9 (12.2, 22.9)‡
25.0–29.9	30.5 (22.4, 40.1)	34.8 (29.6, 40.3)	25.3 (20.1, 31.3)	31.6 (25.9, 37.9)	21.3 (16.5, 27.1)	31.5 (25.8, 37.7)
≥30	58.7 (49.2–67.6)	45.9 (40.2, 51.7)	65.7 (59.8, 71.1)	52.9 (46.4, 59.3)	69.0 (62.6, 74.7)	51.6 (44.5, 58.7)

CI confidence interval

*p<0.01 †p<0.001 across surveys (symbols in column 1 indicate difference with column 1; symbols in column 2 denote difference with column 2; symbols in column 3 indicate difference with column 1)

‡p<0.01, §p<0.001 within survey. Symbols with BP <120/<80 mmHg and BMI <25 kg/m² denote differences in distribution of data for classifying BP and BMI and not only the line indicated

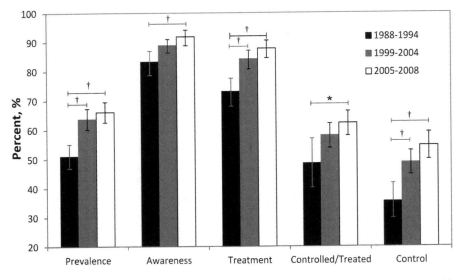

Fig. 1.1 The prevalence, awareness, treatment, and control of hypertension among patients with diabetes mellitus are depicted for three NHANES time periods including 1988–1994, 1999–2004, 2005–2008. *$p<0.01$, †$p<0.001$ between NHANES time periods

diastolic BP generally declined, especially among those who were controlled. Among controlled diabetic hypertensives, BP shifted away from "Stage 2" pre-hypertension (130–139/85–89 mmHg) and toward values in the "Stage 1" and normal range. Among uncontrolled diabetic hypertensives, there was a shift from Stage 2 to Stage 1 hypertension, although the difference was not significant. Body mass index was higher among controlled than uncontrolled diabetic hypertensive patients, although the difference was not statistically significant in 2005–2008.

The clinical epidemiology of hypertension in diabetes (Fig. 1.1). Prevalent hypertension defined as BP ≥140/≥90 mmHg or self-reported hypertension treatment increased from 51% to 66%, $p<0.001$, from 1988–1994 to 2005–2008. During this time period, awareness (83% to 92%, $p<0.001$), treatment (73% to 88%, $p<0.001$), proportion of treated patients controlled (48% to 62%, $p<0.01$), and controlled to <140/<90 mmHg (35.5% to 54.6%, $p<0.001$) all increased.

BP "control" among all diabetic hypertensives (Fig. 1.2). The proportion of all diabetic hypertensives in the three NHANES time periods with BP below various control cut points also increased. The percentage with blood pressure <140/<90 mmHg rose from 35.5% to 54.6% ($p<0.001$), <140/<80 from 28% to 48% ($p<0.001$), <130/85 from 20% to 37% ($p<0.001$), and <130/<80 doubled from 18% to 36% ($p<0.001$).

BP "control" among all patients with diabetes (Fig. 1.3). The proportion of all diabetics in the three NHANES time periods with BP below various levels used to define control increased. The percentage with BP <140/<90 increased from 67% to

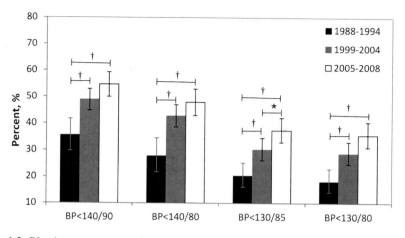

Fig. 1.2 Blood pressure control rates to <140/<90 mmHg, <140/<80, <130/<85, and <130/<80 mmHg are shown for patients with diabetes and hypertension in the three NHANES time periods. *$p < 0.01$, †$p < 0.001$ between NHANES time periods

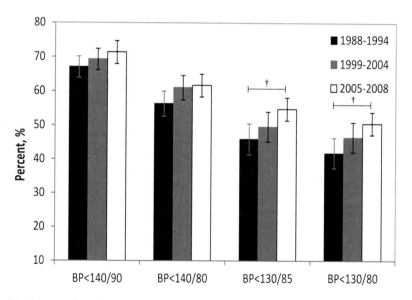

Fig. 1.3 Among all patients with diabetes including those with and without hypertension, the percentages with BP <140/<90 mmHg, <140/<80, <130/<85, and <130/<80 mmHg are shown. *$p < 0.01$, †$p < 0.001$ between NHANES time periods

71% ($p = 0.029$), <140/<80 from 56% to 62% ($p = 0.015$), <130/<85 from 46% to 55% ($p < 0.001$), and <130/<80 from 42% to 50% ($p < 0.001$).

Number of antihypertensive medications reported by diabetic hypertensives (Fig. 1.4). Among all diabetic hypertensives, the percentage untreated declined

Fig. 1.4 The percentage of patients on 0 (untreated), 1, 2, and ≥3 antihypertensive medications are shown for four groups of diabetic hypertensive patients: (**a**) all (**b**) all uncontrolled (**c**) treated uncontrolled (**d**) treated controlled. As noted, some patients who reported taking antihypertensive medications did not bring any or identify any during the examination including "unidentified"

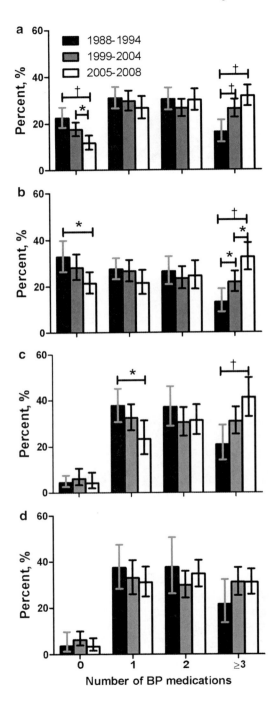

from 22% to 12% ($p < 0.001$), the percentage reporting 1 and 2 medications did not change, and those reporting ≥3 increased ($p < 0.001$, panel a). Among all uncontrolled diabetic hypertensives, the untreated proportion declined from 33% to 21% ($p < 0.01$), and the proportion reporting ≥3 BP medications rose from 13% to 33% ($p < 0.001$, panel b). For the treated, uncontrolled diabetic hypertensives (panel c), 4–6% did not identify any BP medication including "unspecified," despite the fact that they responded affirmatively that they were taking medication to lower BP. Among the treated uncontrolled group, the proportion reporting one BP medication declined from 38% to 23% ($p < 0.01$), while the proportion reporting ≥3 medications increased from 21% to 41% ($p < 0.001$). For treated, controlled diabetic hypertensives, 4–6% did not identify any BP medications, although they responded affirmatively to a question about taking medication to lower BP. In the treated controlled group, the proportion reporting one medication declined, whereas the percentage reporting ≥3 increased. These differences were not statistically significant.

Discussion

Prevalent hypertension among diabetics is approximately double that of nondiabetics and concomitant hypertension increases risk 1.5–3.0-fold further. Treatment of hypertension in diabetics attenuates risk [3–7]. In Syst-Eur, diabetics with Stage 2 isolated systolic hypertension, i.e., systolic BP ≥160 mmHg with normal diastolic BP, had 69% fewer CV events and 76% fewer CV deaths when randomized to nitrendipine than placebo [18]. In the HOT Study, diabetic hypertensives had ~50% fewer CV events when randomized to a diastolic BP of <80 than <90 mmHg [19]. In UKPDS, BP control to 144/82 versus 154/87 mmHg was associated with reductions of a 24% in any diabetes endpoint, 44% in stroke, and 37% in microvascular events [20]. In ADVANCE, reducing BP from 145/81, which is nearly identical to the intensive group in UKPDS, to 136/73, led to reductions of 14% in all cause mortality and coronary events, 18% in CV mortality, and 21% in renal events [21].

In ACCORD, diabetic hypertensives were randomly assigned to target systolic BP <140 versus <120 mmHg [14]. The "less intensive" target led to a mean BP of 133.5/70.5, which is slightly lower than the more intensively treated group in ADVANCE [21]. The more intensively treated group in ACCORD achieved a mean BP of 119.3/64.4. The 14/6 mmHg lower BP was associated with a 12% ($p = 0.20$) reduction in the primary outcome. Collectively, studies suggest that much of the benefit of antihypertensive therapy in diabetics is achieved when systolic BP is reduced to <140 and diastolic BP to <80 mmHg.

Given the prevalence of hypertension in diabetic patients, the adverse effects of hypertension on outcomes, and the benefits of hypertension control, BP management in diabetics has attention in several guidelines and quality improvement programs [8–10]. Our report summarizes the clinical epidemiology of hypertension among diabetics in NHANES.

Prevalence. Prevalent hypertension in adult diabetics increased from 51% in 1988–1994 to 66% in 2005–2008, which is higher than the 57.3% reported previously (Fig. 1.1) [2]. The reason for the discrepancy is unclear, although there were differences in defining diabetes. Prevalent hypertension among all U.S. adults increased from 23.9% in 1988–1994 to 29.0% in 2005–2008 [13]. Thus, prevalent hypertension in diabetics is roughly double than that in nondiabetics. Diabetics are probably more likely than their non-diabetic counterparts to receive antihypertensive treatment when BP is <140 mmHg. Thus, the greater absolute increase in prevalent hypertension in diabetics (51–66% [15%]) than all adults (23.9–29.0% [5%]), may be partially explained by initiation of antihypertensive treatment in diabetics with BP <140/<90.

Awareness. Among diabetic hypertensives, awareness rose from 83% in 1988–1994, to 92% in 2005–2008. Among all hypertensives, awareness rose from 69% to 81% over the same time period [13]. The greater awareness of hypertension among diabetic than all hypertensive patients probably reflects greater emphasis on detection, treatment, and control and more frequent healthcare visits among diabetics than nondiabetics.

Treatment. Among all diabetic hypertensives, 73% were treated in 1988–1994 and rose to 87% in 2005–2008. The percentage of aware diabetic hypertensives on treatment rose from 88% in 1988–1994 (0.73/0.83) to ~95% in 2005–2008. For comparison purposes, among all adult hypertensives, 78% of the aware group were treated in 1988–1994 and nearly 90% in 2005–2008 [13]. Thus, time trends for both diabetic and all hypertensive patients indicate a greater proportion of adults who are aware and reporting treatment. The findings suggest that inertia to beginning pharmacotherapy has declined [14].

Proportion of treated patients controlled. Among adult diabetic hypertensives, the proportion of treated patients controlled to BP <140/<90 mmHg rose from 48% in 1988–1994 to 62% in 2005–2008 (Fig. 1.1). Comparable figures for BP control to <140/<90 among all adult hypertensives were 54% and 69%, respectively [13]. These data are consistent with evidence linking diabetes mellitus to treatment-resistant hypertension [21].

Hypertension control. Among all diabetic hypertensives, BP control to <140/<90 rose from 33.5% in 1988–1994 to 54.6% in 2005–2008. Hypertension control among diabetics are somewhat, but probably not significantly, higher than for all hypertensives of 27.3% in 1988–1994 to 50.1% in 2007–2008 [13].

Since different BP control goals have been published, BP control to <140/<80, <130/<85 and <130/<80 mmHg are also of interest (Fig. 1.2) [8–10, 22]. BP control to all levels improved with time. More improvement was generally observed between 1988–1994 and 1999–2004 than 1999–2004 and 2005–2008 (Fig. 1.1). Given the relatively wide pulse pressure and low diastolic BP in diabetic hypertensives, the similar control rates to <130/<85 and <130/<80 are not surprising. This observation is consistent with the notion that systolic BP control will usually result in diastolic BP control in diabetic hypertensives.

NCQA and PQRI(s) indicators for BP control in diabetes are calculated including all eligible diabetic patients and not just those with hypertension [23, 24]. Not surprisingly, the percentages attaining BP below the various thresholds are greater for all diabetics than for hypertensive diabetics. While the trends are similar, the absolute percentage improvement is somewhat less for all diabetic patients than for the hypertensive diabetic subset alone.

Changes in BP and stages of BP. Blood pressure among diabetic hypertensives declined from 145.2/74.7 mmHg in 1988–1994 to 136.5/69.7 in 2005–2008 (Table 1.2). Comparable data for all hypertensives document that BP fell from 143.0/80.4 to 135.2/74.1 [13]. Thus, systolic BP values were similar, whereas diastolic BP values were lower in diabetic than all hypertensive patients. In diabetic and all hypertensive patients, the decline of BP with time is most likely explained by increases in awareness, treatment, and proportion of treated patients controlled [13]. It is unlikely that lifestyle changes played a major role, since diabetic and all hypertensive patients became more obese [25]. Evidence suggests that dietary patterns also deteriorated with time and became less "DASH-like" [26].

The decline of BP among all diabetic hypertensives, especially systolic BP, was not reflected in comparable changes of BP with time in controlled and uncontrolled diabetic hypertensives separately. Thus, the principal contributor to the decline of systolic BP was the improvement in hypertension control with time. Even in 1988–1994, BP in controlled diabetic hypertensives was ~123/71 and improved modestly to 121/66 in 2005–2008. Among uncontrolled diabetic hypertensives, BP declined modestly from 157/77 to 155/74.

The decline of BP among all diabetic hypertensives was paralleled by an improvement in BP stage, i.e., the percentage with normal BP and "Stage 1" pre-hypertension rose, whereas the percentage with Stage 1 and Stage 2 hypertension declined (Table 1.1). While the BP stage showed some numerical improvement in controlled and uncontrolled diabetic hypertensives separately, the changes were not significant at $p < 0.01$.

Changes in pharmacotherapy and apparent treatment resistant hypertension (Fig. 1.4). Among all diabetic hypertensives, the proportion who were untreated fell from 22% to 12%, while those reportedly taking ≥3 BP medications rose from 16% to 32% (panel a). The term apparent treatment resistant was used to describe this group, since data on medication adherence and BP measurement artifacts are not available in NHANES data [13]. By absolute percentages, more diabetic hypertensives reported taking ≥3 than either one or two BP medications, although differences were not significant.

Among all uncontrolled patients, untreated hypertension declined from 35% to 21%, while the percentage on ≥3 BP medications rose from 13% to 33% (panel b). In treated, uncontrolled diabetic hypertensives, the percentage on one medication fell from 38% to 23%, and the percentage on ≥3 BP medications rose from 21% to 41%, i.e., apparent treatment-resistant hypertension. The number of BP medications reported by treated, controlled diabetic hypertensives did not change significantly with time. Overall, controlled and uncontrolled hypertensive patients are not distinguished by the number of BP medications reported. Of note, 4–6% of treated uncontrolled and controlled patients who reported taking BP medications did not bring any or report any including undefined antihypertensive during examination, which parallels all hypertensives [15]. Limitations of reports on the clinical epidemiology of hypertension from NHANES were noted [13, 15].

Summary. This update on the clinical epidemiology of hypertension in diabetes shows that hypertension awareness, treatment, proportion of treated patients controlled, and controlled have all improved with time. Unfortunately, prevalent hypertension also increased. Our findings have important implications for healthcare policy and practice to further improve the clinical epidemiology of hypertension in diabetics. First, by definition all unaware hypertensives are uncontrolled; 21% of all uncontrolled diabetic hypertensives were untreated and roughly 18% of all uncontrolled hypertensives were unaware in 2005–2008 (0.08 unaware/0.454 uncontrolled=0.18). Thus, ~90% of untreated diabetic hypertensives are unaware. While hypertension awareness is high among diabetics at 92%, further efforts to increase awareness are important in reducing untreated, uncontrolled hypertension in diabetics. Second, 46% of uncontrolled diabetic hypertensives in 2005–2008 reported taking one or two BP medications. Programs to successfully reduce therapeutic inertia should improve BP control in this group [15, 27, 28]. Third, a growing proportion of all treated uncontrolled diabetic hypertensives reports taking ≥3 BP medications and is apparent treatment resistant. Evidence suggests that out-of-office BP monitoring could identify ~35–40% with "office"-resistant hypertension [29]. After identifying "office" resistance and nonadherence, roughly 20–25% of all treated, uncontrolled diabetic hypertensive patients probably are treatment resistant [21, 29]. For this group, comparative effectiveness research is needed to identify the most promising evidence-based interventions for improving BP control [30–33]. The role of catheter-based interventions deserves further study in diabetic hypertensives that remain uncontrolled after exhausting known evidence-based interventions [34, 35]. Last, but certainly not least, public health initiatives to encourage healthy nutrition, physical activity, and adherence with evidence-based treatments could also lower BP and improve control for all hypertensive patients including diabetics [13, 15, 28].

References

1. Salanitro AH, Roimie CL. Blood pressure management in patients with diabetes. Clin Diab. 2010;26:107–14.
2. Keenan NL, Rosendorf KA. Prevalence of hypertension and controlled hypertension—United States, 2005–2008. MMWR. 2011;60:94–7.
3. Kannel WB, McGee DL. Diabetes and cardiovascular disease. J Am Med Assoc. 1979;241:2035–8.
4. Turner RC, Millns H, Neil HAW, Stratton IM, Manley SE, Matthews DR, et al. Risk factors for coronary heart disease in non-insulin dependent diabetes mellitus: United Kingdom prospective diabetes study (UKPDS: 23). Br Med J. 1998;316:823–8.

5. Wilson PWF, D'Agostino RB, Levy D, Belanger AM, Silbershatz H, Kannel WB. Prediction of coronary heart disease using risk factor categories. Circulation. 1998;97:1837–47.
6. Sowers JR, Epstein M, Frohlich ED. Diabetes, hypertension, and cardiovascular disease: an update. Hypertension. 2001;37:1053–9.
7. Wannamethee SG, Shaper AG, Whincup PH, Lennon L, Satar N. Impact of diabetes on cardiovascular disease risk and all-cause mortality in older men. Arch Intern Med. 2011;171:404–10.
8. Bakris GL, Williams M, Dworkin L, Elliott WJ, Epstein M, Toto R, et al. Preserving renal function in adults with hypertension and diabetes: a concensus approach. National Kidney Foundation Hypertension and Diabetes Executive Committee Working Group. Am J Kidney Dis. 2000;36:646–61.
9. Chobanian AV, Bakris GL, Black HR, Cushman WC, Green LA, Izzo JL, et al. Seventh report of the Joint National Committee on prevention, detection, evaluation, and treatment of high blood pressure. Hypertension. 2003;42:1206–52.
10. American Diabetes Association. Standards of medical care in diabetes–2011. Diab Care. 2011;34 Suppl 1:S11–61.
11. Hajjar I, Kotchen TA. Trends in prevalence, awareness, treatment, and control of hypertension in the United States, 1988–2000. J Am Med Assoc. 2003;290:199–206.
12. Ong KL, Cheung BMY, Man YB, Lau CP, Lam KSL. Prevalence, awareness, treatment, and control of hypertension among United States adults 1999–2004. Hypertension. 2007;49:69–75.
13. Egan BM, Zhao Y, Axon RN. US trends in prevalence, awareness, treatment, and control of hypertension, 1988–2008. J Am Med Assoc. 2010;303:2043–50.
14. The Accord Study Group. Effects of intensive blood-pressure control in type 2 diabetes mellitus. N Engl J Med. 2010;362:1575–85.
15. Egan BM, Zhao Y, Axon RN, Brzezinski WA, Ferdinand KC. Uncontrolled and apparent treatment resistant hypertension in the U.S. 1988–2008. Circulation. 2011;124:1046–1058.
16. National Center for Health Statistics. Analytic and reporting guidelines: the Third National Health and Nutrition Examination Survey, NHANES III (1988–94). http://www.cdc.gov/nchs/data/nhanes/nhanes3/nh3gui.pdf. Accessed 29 July 2011.
17. The National Center for Health Statistics. Analytic and reporting guidelines: the National Health and Nutrition Examination Survey. http://www.cdc.gov/nchs/data/ nhanes/ nhanes_03_04/nhanes_analytic _guidelines_dec_2005.pdf. Accessed 29 July 2010.
18. Tuomilehto J, Rastenyte D, Birkenhäger WH, Thijs L, Antikainen J, Bulpitt CJ, et al. Effects of calcium-channel blockade in older patients with diabetes and systolic hypertension. Systolic hypertension in Europe trial investigators. N Engl J Med. 1999;340:677–84.
19. Hansson L, Zanchetti A, Carruthers SG, Dahlöf B, Elmfeldt D, Julius S, et al. Effects of intensive blood-pressure lowering and low-dose aspirin in patients with hypertension: principal results of the hypertension optimal treatment (HOT) randomised trial. HOT study group. Lancet. 1998;13(351):1755–62.
20. UK Prospective Diabetes Study Group. Tight blood pressure control and risk of macrovascular and microvascular complications in type 2 diabetes: UKPDS 38. Br Med J. 1998;317:703–13.
21. Calhoun DA, Jones D, Textor S, Goff DC, Murphy TP, Toto RD, et al. Resistant hypertension: diagnosis, evaluation, and treatment: a scientific statement from the American Heart Association Professional Education Committee of the Council for High Blood Pressure Research. Hypertension. 2008;51:1403–19.
22. Quinn RR, Hemmelgarn BR, Padwal RS, Myers MG, Cloutier L, Bolli P, et al. The 2010 Canadian Hypertension Education Program recommendations for the management of hypertension: part I—blood pressure measurement, diagnosis and assessment of risk. Can J Cardiol. 2010;26:241–8.
23. National Center for Quality Assurance HEDIS®. Technical specifications for physician measurement. Compr diabetes care. 2011;pp. 154–166.
24. https://www.cms.gov/PQRS/15_MeasuresCodes.asp. Accessed 5 Aug 2011.

25. Mellen PB, Gao SK, Vitolins MZ, Goff DC. Deteriorating dietary habits among adults with hypertension. Arch Intern Med. 2008;168:308–14.
26. Ford ES, Zhao G, Li C, Pearson WS, Mokdad AH. Trends in obesity and abdominal obesity among hypertensive and nonhypertensive adults in the United States. Am J Hypertens. 2008;21:1124–8.
27. Okonofua EC, Simpson K, Jesri A, Rehman S, Durkalski V, Egan BM. Therapeutic inertia is an impediment to achieving the Healthy People 2010 blood pressure control goals. Hypertension. 2006;47:1–7.
28. Egan BM, Laken MA. Is BP control to <140/<90 mmHg in 50% of all hypertensive patients as good as we can do in the United States? Or is this as good as it gets? Curr Opin Cardiol. 2011;26:356–61.
29. de la Sierra A, Segura J, Banegas JR, Gorostidi M, de la Cruz JJ, Armario P, et al. Clinical features of 8295 patients with resistant hypertension classified on the basis of ambulatory blood pressure monitoring. Hypertension. 2011;57:898–902.
30. Pimenta E, Calhoun DA. Resistant hypertension and aldosteronism. Curr Hypertens Rep. 2007;9:353–9.
31. Taler SJ, Textor SC, Augustine JE. Resistant hypertension: comparing hemodynamic management to specialist care. Hypertension. 2002;39:982–8.
32. Egan BM, Basile JN, Rehman SU, Strange P, Grob C, Riehle J, et al. Renin-guided algorithm matches clinical hypertension specialist care in uncontrolled hypertension: A randomized-controlled clinical trial. Am J Hypertens. 2009;22:792–801.
33. Mann SJ. Drug therapy for resistant hypertension: simplifying the approach. J Clin Hypertens. 2011;13:120–30.
34. Symplicity HTN–2 Investigators. Renal sympathetic denervation in patients with treatment-resistant hypertension (the simplicity HTN-2 trial): a randomized controlled trial. Lancet. 2010;376:1903–9.
35. Wustmann K, Kucera JP, Scheffers I, Mohaupt M, Kroon AA, Leeuw PW, et al. Effects of chronic baroreceptor stimulation on the autonomic cardiovascular regulation in patients with drug-resistant arterial hypertension. Hypertension. 2009;54:530–6.

Chapter 2
Evaluation and Management of Secondary Hypertension

Nathaniel Winer

Introduction

Most patients who present with elevated blood pressure (BP) will have essential (idiopathic) hypertension; extensive laboratory evaluation for secondary causes in these patients is low-yield and cost-prohibitive. However, identification of a secondary cause may often lead to a cure of the elevated BP or to a decrease in the number and/or doses of antihypertensive agents and a reduction in the long-term cardiovascular risks of hypertension. This chapter will focus on two important causes of secondary hypertension: renovascular stenosis and primary aldosteronism. Other causes of secondary hypertension include primary renal disease, oral contraceptive use, pheochromocytoma, Cushing's syndrome, sleep apnea syndrome, and coarctation of the aorta. Clinical features which are suggestive of these disorders are given in Table 2.1.

Secondary hypertension should be suspected in the following conditions: severe or resistant hypertension; acute BP elevation in a medication-adherent patient with preceding stable hypertension; a history of prepubertal onset hypertension; young nonobese, white patients without risk factors, such as diabetes, chronic kidney disease, or a family history of hypertension; and malignant hypertension (severe hypertension associated with acute renal failure, retinal hemorrhages, papilledema, and neurologic findings).

N. Winer, M.D. (✉)
Department of Medicine, Division of Endocrinology, SUNY Downstate Medical Center,
Brooklyn, NY 11203, USA
e-mail: Nathaniel.winer@downstate.edu

S.I. McFarlane and G.L. Bakris (eds.), *Diabetes and Hypertension: Evaluation and Management*, Contemporary Diabetes, DOI 10.1007/978-1-60327-357-2_2,
© Springer Science+Business Media New York 2012

Table 2.1 Other causes of secondary hypertension

Disorder	Suggestive clinical features
Primary renal disease	↑ Serum creatinine, abnormal urinalysis
Oral contraceptives	New-onset hypertension related to BCP use
Pheochromocytoma	Paroxysmal BP spikes, headaches, sweats, tachycardia
Cushing's syndrome	Moon facies, central obesity, striae, hirsutism, ↑ BP, ↑ glucose
Sleep apnea syndrome	Male obesity, loud snoring, daytime somnolence
Coarctation of aorta	↑ BP in arms, ↓ femoral pulses, ↓ BP in legs
Hypothyroidism	Symptoms of hypothyroidism, ↑ TSH, ↓ Free T4
1° hyperparathyroidism	Hypercalcemia, ↑ PTH

Causes of Secondary Hypertension

Renovascular Hypertension

Prevalence

Although renovascular stenosis is a common and progressive disease in patients with atherosclerosis, it is a relatively uncommon cause of hypertension in patients with mild hypertension. Of 834 individuals ≥65 years old who underwent renal artery duplex ultrasound as part of their cardiovascular health study, the overall prevalence rate of significant renovascular disease was 6.8% [1]. In contrast, renal artery stenosis is more frequent in certain high-risk populations. For example, renovascular stenosis was seen in 30% of patients undergoing screening renal artery angiography at the time of cardiac catheterization [2], in 22–59% of patients with carotid artery and peripheral vascular disease [3], and in 10–45% of white patients with severe or malignant hypertension [4]. Nonwhite patients with severe or malignant hypertension are more likely to have essential hypertension.

Pathophysiology

About 90% of all renal stenotic lesions are due to atherosclerosis, which often accompanies systemic atherosclerosis that involves the aortic, coronary, cerebral, or peripheral arteries. Fibromuscular dysplasia (FMD) is the second most common cause of renal artery stenosis and most frequently affects young women, although FMD can occur in either gender at any age.

Clinical Cues

Findings that suggest renovascular stenosis are onset of BP <160/100 mmHg after 55 years of age; a 25% or greater rise in serum creatinine after institution of an ACE

Table 2.2 Clinical clues to diagnosis of renovascular hypertension[a]

Onset of hypertension before 30 years or severe hypertension after 55 year

Accelerated, malignant, or resistant hypertension

New-onset azotemia or worsening renal function after ACE/ARB Rx

Unexplained atrophic kidney or difference in kidney size >1.5 cm

Sudden, unexplained pulmonary edema

Abdominal systolic diastolic bruit

Multivessel coronary artery disease

Unexplained congestive heart failure

Refractory angina

[a]Adapted from [6]

inhibitor or angiotensin II receptor blocker; moderate or severe hypertension in a patient with a kidney <9 cm in length or a >1.5 cm difference in renal size; recurrent episodes of flash pulmonary edema, resolved by angioplasty or surgical treatment [5]; and an abdominal systolic–diastolic bruit (found in 40% of patients) (Table 2.2). Radiographic studies should be undertaken if clinical history and physical findings are suggestive of renal artery stenosis, BP uncontrolled despite optimal doses of antihypertensive medications, and the patient agrees to undergo remedial procedures.

Primary Diagnostic Tests

Although renal angiography remains the gold standard for diagnosing renal artery stenosis, less invasive alternative screening procedures such as magnetic resonance angiography (MRA), computed tomographic angiography (CTA), and Duplex Doppler ultrasonography may be appropriate initial steps. However, if findings are inconclusive with these methods, and clinical suspicion is high, renal angiography may be required. MRA is highly sensitive in patients who have clinical characteristics of renal artery stenosis except in those who are likely to have fibromuscular disease, which typically affects the distal two-thirds of the renal artery and its branches, in contrast to atherosclerotic disease which usually involves the ostium and proximal one-third of the main renal artery and the perirenal aorta [7]. The sensitivity and specificity of CTA for detecting stenoses >50% and lesions in the main renal artery is over 90%. Duplex Doppler ultrasonography, which directly visualizes the renal arteries via B-mode imaging and compares the systolic flow velocity in the aorta with that in the renal artery via Doppler, can identify a narrowed artery segment by an increase in flow velocity. In a meta-analysis of 88 studies of 9,974 arteries in 8,147 patients, peak systolic velocity was more accurate than renal-aortic ratio peak systolic velocity, showing a sensitivity of 85% and specificity of 92% [8]. The method has the advantage of being able to detect both unilateral and bilateral renal artery disease, but is time consuming to perform, has a steep learning curve, and is highly operator dependant.

Ancillary Diagnostic Tests

Selective renal vein renin measurements, plasma renin activity, and renal scintigraphy are not helpful screening tests because of poor sensitivity and specificity, and the need to discontinue antihypertensive agents, including ACE inhibitors, angiotensin II receptor blockers, β-blockers, and diuretics, which may affect plasma renin activity. However, if captopril, 25–50 mg, is administered 1 h prior to the renal scan, blockade of the angiotensin II-mediated decline in GFR in the affected kidney, and an accompanying increase in GFR in the contralateral kidney, may decrease or delay the uptake, or slow the washout of radiolabeled DPTA, hippurate, or MAG3 in the stenotic kidney. Thus, captopril renal scintigraphy may be useful in screening for renovascular stenosis in patients at high risk for renovascular stenosis and in evaluating the hemodynamic significance of a stenotic lesion [6].

Treatment

Medical therapy with agents that block the renin-angiotensin system (ACE inhibitors and angiotensin II blockers) has been effective in BP control [9]; thiazide diuretics (especially chlorthalidone), calcium channel blockers, and β-blockers may be added, if needed. With medical therapy there is a risk that progression of the stenosis may occur [10]; however, concomitant treatment of dyslipidemia and effective glycemic control in patients with diabetes may mitigate progression of atherosclerosis. Worsening kidney failure during medical therapy appears to be unlikely in unilateral renal artery stenosis [11], but in patients with bilateral renal artery stenosis or stenosis in a solitary functioning kidney deterioration of renal function and mortality risk are greater [12].

Revascularization may be indicated in patients with hemodynamically significant lesions who meet the criteria listed in Table 2.2. The procedure of choice in most centers is percutaneous transluminal angioplasty with stent implantation, particularly with proximal artery or ostial disease [6, 13]. Surgical revascularization would be indicated if angioplasty fails or with multiple small arteries, early branching of the main renal artery, or with coexisting aortic aneurysm or severe aortoiliac disease [6].

Primary Aldosteronism

Pathophysiology

The two major secretogogues for aldosterone are angiotensin II (AII) and serum K+ levels. AII signals adrenal glomerulosa cells via G-protein-coupled receptors, which activate K+ channels to set glomerulosa cell resting membrane potential. Both AII signaling and increased extracellular K+ cause cell membrane depolarization leading to activation of voltage-gated Ca++ channels. Increased intracellular Ca++, in turn, stimulates expression of enzymes, such as aldosterone synthase, which are

Table 2.3 Subtypes of PA (% of cases)		
•	Bilateral adrenal hyperplasia (IHA)	(60%)
•	Aldosterone-producing adenoma (APA)	(35%)
•	Unilateral adrenal hyperplasia	(2%)
•	Aldosterone-producing adrenocortical carcinoma	(<1%)
•	Glucocorticoid-remediable aldosteronism (GRA)	(<1%)
•	Ectopic aldosterone-producing adenoma/carcinoma	(<1%)
•	Familial hyperaldosteronism (FH type II)	?

required for aldosterone production and also produces glomerulosa cell proliferation. Recently, two loss of function mutations in the gene, KCNJ5, which encodes the glomerulosa cell K+ channel, have been identified in aldosterone-producing adrenal tumors in 8 of 22 patients with primary aldosteronism and a third mutation was found in a father and two daughters with massive adrenal hyperplasia [14]. Excessive aldosterone secretion promotes renal tubular sodium reabsorption, renal K+ loss, extracellular volume expansion, and hypertension, findings which characterize classical primary aldosteronism (Conn's syndrome).

Subtypes of PA

The most common subtypes of PA are bilateral adrenal hyperplasia (idiopathic hyperaldosteronism or IHA) and unilateral aldosterone-producing adenoma (APA). Less common varieties are given in Table 2.3. Primary adrenal hyperplasia (PAH), characterized by predominantly unilateral micro- or macro-nodular hyperplasia of the adrenal glomerulosa, and adrenal cortical carcinoma are relatively rare causes of PA. Glucocorticoid remediable aldosteronism (GRA, dexamethasone-suppressible hyperaldosteronism, or familial hyperaldosteronism, type I) is a rare, dominantly inherited form of PA, often found in early childhood or adolescence, and associated with an increased incidence of cerebral aneurysms. The disorder results from a "chimeric" gene whose product (located ectopically in the adrenal fasciculata) has actions of both aldosterone synthase and 11β-hydroxylase. In GRA aldosterone secretion is regulated by ACTH, rather than by angiotensin II. Consequently, aldosterone secretion parallels the diurnal variation of ACTH rather than changes in sodium balance, resulting in chronic mineralocorticoid excess and hypertension. Genetic testing of peripheral blood leucocyte DNA is a highly sensitive and specific method for diagnosing GRA [15]. Familial hyperaldosteronism (FH II) due to either IHA or APA is reported to be more common than GRA, but its genetic basis remains to be determined.

The prevalence of PA increases with the degree of hypertension and with resistant hypertension [16]. Patients with PA are at greater risk for cardiovascular events compared to those with comparable blood pressure levels. PA is also associated with increased arterial wall thickness, central artery stiffness, and albumin excretion compared to age-matched controls. Blocking the actions of aldosterone with spironolactone improves survival in older persons with congestive heart failure.

Diagnosis of PA

Screening for PA

Since the introduction of plasma aldosterone:plasma renin activity (PAC:PRA) ratio in 1981 the prevalence rate of PA has increased from <0.5% to the current 4.6–13% [17]. Newly diagnosed cases have increased more than tenfold; the proportion of IHA cases has risen from 40% to 60%, while APA cases have declined from >70% to 35%; concurrently, the incidence of hypokalemia has decreased from ≥80% to ≤20%.

The morning PAC:PRA ratio has >90% sensitivity and specificity. PAC:PRA is unaffected by posture and antihypertensive drugs, except for amiloride (Midamor) and the mineralocorticoid receptor antagonists, spironolactone (Aldactone) and eplerenone (Inspra), which must be discontinued for at least 6 weeks prior to testing. Angiotensin-converting enzyme inhibitors, angiotensin receptor blockers, and diuretics can be continued; because these agents stimulate renin secretion, suppressed PRA makes underlying PA more likely. Inappropriate elevation of PAC in the face of suppression of renin secretion by adrenergic blockade with β-blockers or central α_2-agonists is consistent with PA. In hypokalemic subjects raising serum potassium levels into the mid-normal range with potassium supplementation will increase PAC and optimize the PAC:PRA ratio. Table 2.4 lists clinical settings in which screening should be performed in patients with hypertension.

Confirming PA

Techniques to confirm the diagnosis of PA rely on evaluating the effect of volume expansion on the suppressibility of PAC or urinary aldosterone. These consist of:

1. *Oral Salt-loading*. Patients whose hypertension and hypokalemia have been controlled are placed on a high sodium diet for 3 days and given supplementary sodium chloride tablets to achieve a sodium excretion >200 mmol per day. Since high dietary sodium intake may increase potassium excretion, serum potassium must be monitored and replaced as needed. On day 3 aldosterone ≥12 μg and sodium ≥200 mmol in a 24-h urine collection indicate autonomous adrenal function.

2. *Intravenous saline infusion*. Unlike normal subjects patients with PA fail to show suppression of PAC with saline infusion. After overnight fasting 2 L of normal saline are infused over a 4-h period. Preexisting left ventricular dysfunction or renal dysfunction may increase the risk for acute volume overload. Postinfusion PAC in normal subjects is <5 μg/dL, whereas patients with PA do not suppress below 10 ng/dL. Patients with IHA may have PAC between 5 and 10 ng/dL.

3. *Fludrocortisone suppression*. Fludrocortisone acetate (Florinef), 0.1 mg every 6 h for 4 days, is given with sodium chloride, 2 g three times daily with meals,

Table 2.4 Indications to screen for PA

- Hypertension and hypokalemia, spontaneous or diuretic induced
- Resistant hypertension
- Blood pressure: systolic ≥160 or diastolic ≥100 mmHg
- Juvenile hypertension
- Family history of early onset hypertension/hemorrhagic strokes
- Adrenal incidentaloma

while monitoring BP and serum K+ daily. Confirmation of PA requires morning upright PAC to be ≥6 ng/dL on day 4. The association of QT dispersion and left ventricular dysfunction with fludrocortisone testing has discouraged its use.

Determining Subtype

Subtype diagnosis is critical because unilateral adrenalectomy will correct hypokalemia and improve or normalize blood pressure in up to 60% of patients with APA or PAH, whereas surgery in IHA or GRA is usually ineffective and necessitates lifetime adrenal corticoid replacement therapy.

Adrenal CT scan. In a patient <40 years old with PA and a 1–2 cm, unilateral, hypodense, single adenoma, unilateral adrenalectomy should be considered, since nonfunctioning "incidental" adrenal masses are less common in younger patients. However, because adrenal CT often fails to reveal adenomas <1 cm, or may show small bilateral macro- or micro-adenomas, minimal thickening of adrenal limbs, or nonfunctioning adrenal masses in older persons, further testing may be indicated. Patients with "high probability APA" are likely to be younger, more hypertensive, more often hypokalemic, and have higher aldosterone levels than those with IHA.

Adrenal vein sampling. Because adrenal CT lacks reliability in differentiating APA from IHA, adrenal vein sampling is necessary in patients who have high probability APA and seek potential surgical cure of hypertension. Aldosterone and cortisol are measured in blood samples obtained from the adrenal veins and inferior vena cava (IVC). Cosyntropin (Cortrosyn) infusion stabilizes cortisol secretion, maximizes the adrenal vein/IVC cortisol gradient, and stimulates aldosterone secretion from an adenoma. A post-cosyntropin adrenal vein/IVC cortisol ratio ≥10:1 confirms appropriate catheter positioning. Since cortisol secretion is similar from each adrenal the aldosterone/cortisol (A/C ratio) serves as a marker of the dilution of the aldosterone concentration by venous blood. Adrenal vein A/C: ratios ≥4:1 (affected vs. contralateral adrenal) are consistent with unilateral aldosterone excess (APA or PAH), whereas ratios ≤3:1 indicate bilateral aldosterone hypersecretion. Because the right adrenal vein is short and angles superiorly, angiographers inexperienced in adrenal vein catheterization may be unsuccessful in cannulating the right adrenal vein. However, in the absence of a right adrenal vein sample, if the left adrenal vein A/C ratio is significantly lower than that of the IVC, a right adrenal source of the aldosterone excess is likely [19]. Pharmacologic treatment should be

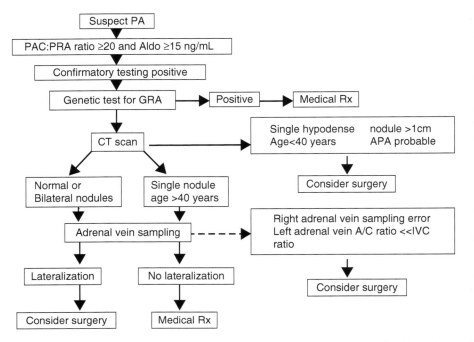

Fig. 2.1 Algorithm for adrenal vein sampling. Young patients (age <20 years) with positive screening and confirmatory tests for hyperaldosteronism should have a genetic test for glucocorticoid-remediable aldosteronism (GRA) if there is a family of hypertension and hemorrhagic strokes. Laparoscopic excision of the adrenal should be considered if CT scan shows a single hypodense nodule >1 cm in persons <40 years of age. Older patients with a unilateral nodule, bilateral nodules, or a normal CT scan require adrenal vein sampling for aldosterone and cortisol. Findings can still be interpreted in the event of failure to obtain a right adrenal vein sample if the inferior vena cava A/C ratio is markedly greater than the left adrenal A/C ratio

considered in clinical settings in which adrenal vein sampling is not available or experience in performing the procedure is lacking. An algorithm showing the diagnostic steps in the differential diagnosis of primary aldosteronism is shown in Fig. 2.1.

[131]I-19-Iodocholesterol adrenal scintigraphy, posture stimulation testing, and measurement of plasma 18-hydroxycorticosterone levels have largely been abandoned because of lack of sensitivity and/or availability.

Treatment

The goal of treatment is not only to normalize elevated blood pressure and hypokalemia, but also to protect against the adverse cardiovascular effects of aldosterone excess.

Surgical treatment of APA or PAH. Unilateral laparoscopic adrenalectomy is preferred over laparotomy because of lower morbidity and shorter hospitalization stays. Preoperative correction of hypokalemia with potassium supplements and/or mineralocorticoid receptor antagonists decreases surgical risk; however, these agents should be withdrawn postoperatively to prevent hyperkalemia. PAC should be determined 1–2 days after surgery to confirm biochemical cure. Short-term fludrocortisone and a liberal sodium intake may be required in the 5% of patients who develop hyperkalemia after surgery.

Pharmacologic treatment. Patients with IHA and GRA and those with APA who are not treated surgically should receive mineralocorticoid receptor antagonists. Traditionally, spironolactone is started at 12.5–25 mg per day and titrated to 400 mg per day, if necessary, to raise serum potassium into the high-normal range without oral potassium supplementation. Normalization of elevated blood pressure may take 1–2 months after which spironolactone can be tapered. Spironolactone, by blocking testosterone receptors and stimulating progesterone receptors, may cause gynecomastia, erectile dysfunction, and decreased libido in men and menstrual abnormalities in women. Eplerenone is a selective mineralocorticoid receptor antagonist which has relatively weak binding affinity for testosterone and progesterone receptors. Because eplerenone has a shorter half-life than spironolactone and may be 25–50% less potent on a weight basis, its starting dose is 25 mg twice daily. Patients with IHA frequently require addition of a thiazide diuretic, since hypervolemia may cause resistance to antihypertensive drug therapy.

Treatment of patients with GRA requires treatment with physiologic doses of a shorter acting glucocorticoid, such as prednisone or hydrocortisone. A mineralocorticoid receptor antagonist may be equally effective and may avoid the potential adverse effects of steroid therapy, especially in children.

References

1. Hansen KJ, Edwards MS, Craven TE, et al. Prevalence of renovascular disease in the elderly: a population-based study. J Vasc Surg. 2002;36:443–51.
2. Harding MB, Smith LR, Himmelstein SI, et al. Renal artery stenosis: prevalence and associated risk factors in patients undergoing routine cardiac catheterization. J Am Soc Nephrol. 1992;2:1608–16.
3. Zierler RE, Bergelin RO, Polissar NL, et al. Carotid and lower extremity arterial disease in patients with renal artery atherosclerosis. Arch Intern Med. 1998;158:761–7.
4. Svetkey LP, Kadir S, Dunnick NR, et al. Similar prevalence of renovascular hypertension in selected blacks and whites. Hypertension. 1991;17:678.
5. Pickering TG, Herman L, Devereux RB, et al. Recurrent pulmonary oedema in hypertension due to bilateral renal artery stenosis: treatment by angioplasty or surgical revascularization. Lancet. 1988;2:551.
6. Hirsch AT, Haskal ZJ, Hertzer NR, et al. ACC/AHA 2005 practice guidelines for the management of patients with peripheral arterial disease (lower extremity, renal, mesenteric, and abdominal aortic): a collaborative report from the American Association for Vascular Surgery/ Society for Vascular Surgery, Society for Cardiovascular Angiography and Interventions,

Society for Vascular Medicine and Biology, Society of Interventional Radiology, and the ACC/AHA task force on practice guidelines (writing committee to develop guidelines for the management of patients with peripheral arterial disease): endorsed by the American Association of Cardiovascular and Pulmonary Rehabilitation; National Heart, Lung, and Blood Institute; Society for Vascular Nursing; TransAtlantic Inter-Society Consensus; and Vascular Disease Foundation. Circulation. 2006;113:e463–654.

7. Safian RD, Textor SC. Renal artery stenosis. N Engl J Med. 2001;344:431–42.
8. Williams GJ, Macaskill P, Chan SF, et al. Comparative accuracy of renal duplex sonographic parameters in the diagnosis of renal artery stenosis: paired and unpaired analysis. Am J Roentgenol. 2007;188:798.
9. Tullis MJ, Caps MT, Zierler RE, et al. Blood pressure, antihypertensive medication, and atherosclerotic renal artery stenosis. Am J Kidney Dis. 1999;33:675.
10. Pohl MA, Novick AC. Natural history of atherosclerotic and fibrous renal artery disease: clinical implications. Am J Kidney Dis. 1985;5:A120.
11. Leertouwer TC, Pattynama PM, van den Berg-Huysmans A. Incidental renal artery stenosis in peripheral vascular disease: a case for treatment? Kidney Int. 2001;59:1480.
12. Chábová V, Schirger A, Stanson AW, et al. Outcomes of atherosclerotic renal artery stenosis managed without revascularization. Mayo Clin Proc. 2000;75:437.
13. van de Ven PJ, Kaatee R, Beutler JJ, et al. Arterial stenting and balloon angioplasty in ostial atherosclerotic renovascular disease: a randomised trial. Lancet. 1999;353:282.
14. Choi M, Scholl UI, Yue P, et al. K+channel mutations in adrenal aldosterone-producing adenomas and hereditary hypertension. Science. 2011;331:768–72.
15. Litchfield WR, Anderson BF, Weiss RJ, et al. Intracranial aneurysm and hemorrhagic stroke in glucocorticoid-remediable aldosteronism. Hypertension. 1998;31:445.
16. Calhoun DA, Nishizaka MK, Zaman MA, et al. Hyperaldosteronism among black and white subjects with resistant hypertension. Hypertension. 2002;40:892.
17. Hiramatsu K, Yamada T, Yukimura Y, et al. A screening test to identify aldosterone-producing adenoma by measuring plasma renin activity. Results in hypertensive patients. Arch Intern Med. 1981;141:1589.
18. Mulatero P, Stowasser M, Loh KC, Fardella CE, et al. Increased diagnosis of primary aldosteronism, including surgically correctable forms, in centers from five continents. J Clin Endocrinol Metab. 2004;89:1045.
19. Young WF, Stanson AW, Thompson GB, et al. Role for adrenal venous sampling in primary aldosteronism. Surgery. 2004;136:1227.

Chapter 3
Hypertension in African Americans

Mahboob Rahman

Introduction

Hypertension is a common clinical problem in African Americans and is associated with significant morbidity and mortality. Though there is a perception that hypertension can be difficult to control in this population, good understanding of the multitude of factors that can influence blood pressure can facilitate better management practices. In this chapter, we summarize the epidemiology and pathophysiology, and outline some strategies for systematic evaluation and management of hypertension in African Americans.

Epidemiology

Hypertension is more common in African-American men (42 %) and women (44%) compared to white men (31%) and women (28%) [1]. African Americans between the ages of 45 and 84 are more than twice as likely as whites to develop incident hypertension [2]. Mortality is higher in black compared to white hypertensive patients, though mortality rates in hypertensive blacks have improved recent years [3].

M. Rahman, M.D., M.S. (✉)
Division of Nephrology and Hypertension, Case Western Reserve University,
11100 Euclid Ave, Cleveland, OH, USA
e-mail: Mahboob.Rahman@uhhospitals.org

S.I. McFarlane and G.L. Bakris (eds.), *Diabetes and Hypertension: Evaluation and Management*, Contemporary Diabetes, DOI 10.1007/978-1-60327-357-2_3,
© Springer Science+Business Media New York 2012

This may relate to inadequate control of blood pressure; non-Hispanic blacks have 90% higher odds of poorly controlled blood pressure compared with non-Hispanic whites after adjustment for sociodemographic and clinical characteristics [4]. According to the recent NHANES data, 71% of African-American hypertensives were being treated, and 42% were being controlled to target blood pressure [1]. This indicates that are opportunities for improvement in initiating treatment, and achieving blood pressure control in African Americans with hypertension. Given the burden of hypertension in this population, this is a task of considerable public health significance.

Pathophysiology

The higher prevalence of hypertension in African Americans is likely related to many different factors. Obesity is more common in African Americans and along with other lifestyle habits such as increased dietary sodium intake (particularly with the higher proclivity to salt sensitivity of blood pressure) and lower dietary potassium intake may contribute to the higher prevalence of hypertension [5–7]. In addition, there are racial differences in sympathetic nervous system activity [8], vascular structure, and function in response to various stimuli that may predispose to development of higher blood pressure and related target organ damage [9].

Hypertensive Target Organ Damage

African Americans with hypertension often develop sequelae of long-standing hypertension. Left ventricular hypertrophy is more common in African Americans than whites. This difference starts at an early age; in young black males, there is a significantly stronger association of LV concentric hypertrophy with BP (systolic BP, odds ratio [OR] 3.74, $p < 0.001$) than whites (systolic BP, OR 1.50, $p = 0.037$). This suggests that elevated BP levels have a greater detrimental effect on LV hypertrophy patterns in the black versus white young adults [10]. Therefore, not surprisingly, incident heart failure is substantially more common among black than nonblack hypertensive patients (5 year incidence rates 7.0% vs. 3.1%, $P < 0.001$). The increased risk of developing new heart failure in blacks persists after adjusting for the higher prevalence of heart failure risk factors in blacks [11].

Chronic kidney disease is an important manifestation of hypertensive target organ damage in African Americans. End-stage renal disease is more common in African Americans than other racial ethnic groups; approximately 30% of patients with end-stage renal disease are African Americans [12]. Hypertensive nephrosclerosis can be the primary cause of renal disease, or hypertension can worsen progression of kidney disease regardless of the etiology of the underlying disease. Interesting new evidence suggests that genetic associations with the MYH9 and apolipoprotein L1 genes may contribute to the higher risk of ESRD in hypertensive African Americans [13]. The prevalence of stroke is higher in African Americans than other racial ethnic groups; this is particularly true in the young African Americans living in the southeastern United States [14]. While many factors contribute to this higher risk, uncontrolled blood pressure represents an important modifiable factor.

Clinical Evaluation

A comprehensive history, physical exam, and basic lab evaluation are recommended for the initial evaluation of all hypertensive patients. The goal of the evaluation is to identify clues suggestive of secondary hypertension, estimate risk of future cardiovascular events, and identify coexistent clinical conditions that affect prognosis and choice of antihypertensive drug therapy and lifestyle factors that influence control of blood pressure.

Accurate measurement of blood pressure is essential for management of hypertension. Standard guidelines for the process of measurement of blood pressure should be followed as carefully as possible [15]. Home and ambulatory blood pressure monitoring are useful adjuncts in the management of hypertension by allowing the identification of white coat (high office and normal out-of-office blood pressure) and masked hypertension (normal office and high out-of-office blood pressure) [16]. This is particularly helpful in African-American patients with hypertensive chronic kidney disease in whom masked hypertension is more common with elevation in nocturnal blood pressure [17].

A thorough medical history should include duration of hypertension, previous experience with antihypertensive drug therapy, symptoms of target organ damage (such as headache, chest pain, shortness of breath), symptoms suggestive of secondary hypertension (paroxysmal headache, flushing labile blood pressure), and intake of over-the-counter medications/herbal products that may influence blood pressure. Careful ascertainment of history of coexistent medical conditions such as diabetes, heart failure, and coronary heart disease is important. Family history of hypertension, particularly at an early age, and presence of kidney failure in other family members provide important prognostic information. Thorough assessment of lifestyle habits as they relate to hypertension such as diet (intake of sodium, potassium saturated fat), exercise habits, weight loss efforts, smoking, alcohol, and illegal drug use can help the clinical guide the patient in developing appropriate interventions.

Physical exam should include fundoscopic evaluation for hypertensive retinopathy and the presence of bruits in the carotid and epigastric areas in addition to a standard thorough cardiovascular examination. Lab evaluation can be limited to a comprehensive metabolic panel, measurement of proteinuria (by albumin/creatinine ratio), and an EKG in most patients. Other tests such as thyroid function, echocardiography, or renal ultrasound may be considered depending on the clinical circumstances.

Treatment Goals in African Americans

The blood pressure treatment target for most hypertensive patients, as recommended by current national guidelines, is <140/90 mmHg [18]. In patients with diabetes and chronic kidney disease, the blood pressure goal is <130/80 mmHg [18].

Recent guidelines from the International Society for Hypertension in Blacks (ISHIB) call for a lower goal; in patients with hypertension and no target organ damage, the recommended goal blood pressure is <135/85 mmHg [6]. In patients with hypertension and target organ damage, preclinical cardiovascular disease, and/ or a history of cardiovascular disease, a goal blood pressure <130/80 mmHg is recommended. These guidelines are based on observational studies and subgroups analyses of clinical trials that support a beneficial effect of lower blood pressure. However, large randomized clinical trials in diabetic patients [19] and patients with chronic kidney disease (with the important exception of patients with proteinuria) [20] have not convincingly demonstrated the benefit of lower than usual reduction of blood pressure. Therefore, other experts have questioned the evidence supporting lower blood pressure goals in African-American patients [21]. The overall approach to blood pressure goals and choices of drug therapy in the ISHIB guidelines is summarized in Fig. 3.1.

Achieving Goals of Therapy

Though it is commonly perceived that blood pressure is difficult to control, several clinical trials have shown that it is feasible to achieve and maintain good blood pressure control in African-American patients with hypertension [22, 23]. In addition to traditional office-based blood pressure management, several novel approaches to improving blood pressure control should be considered. For example, combined home blood pressure monitoring and a tailored behavioral phone intervention reduced systolic blood pressure by 7.5 mmHg compared to usual care in African-American hypertensive patients [24]. Disease management administered by nurses [25], involvement of the patient and the community by culturally appropriate story telling [26], and use of barbers to become health educators, monitor BP, and promote physician follow-up [27] are some innovative ways that have been shown in carefully conducted clinical trials to result in improved blood pressure control. Several community-based programs are currently being evaluated [28].

Physician inertia remains an important barrier; blacks were less likely to have treatment intensified after presenting with uncontrolled blood pressure [29]. Blacks indicated worse medication adherence, more discrimination, and more concerns about high BP and BP medications, compared with whites. These data suggest that it is important that management of hypertension should not simply focus on antihypertensive drug therapy as is often the case in clinical practice, but take into account heath beliefs, experiences with care, and social support [30, 31].

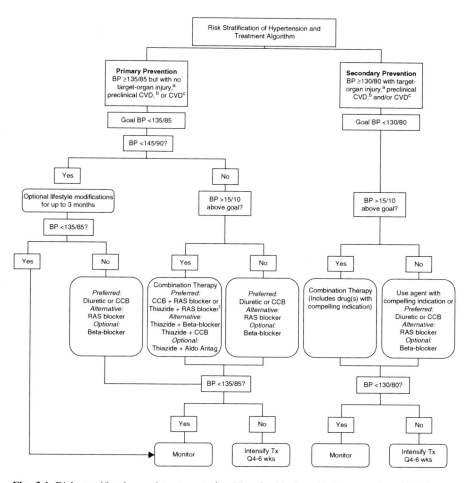

Fig. 3.1 Risk stratification and treatment algorithm for blacks with hypertension. Aldo Antag indicates aldosterone antagonist; Tx, treatment. aTreatment organ damage as albumin:creatinine ratio >200 mg/g, eGFR < 60 mL/min/1.73 m2, or electrocardiographic or electrocardiographic evidence of LVH. bindicators of preclinical include metabolic syndrome, Framingham risk score >20%, prediabetes (impaired fasting glucose [100–125 mg/dL] and/or impaired glucose tolerance [2-hpostload glucose >140 mg/dL]), or diabetes mellitus. cCVD includes HF (systolic or diastolic),CHD/postmyocardial infarction, peripheral arterial disease, stroke, transient ischemic attack, and/ or abdominal aortic aneurysm. Adapted from [6]

Nondrug Therapy

Lifestyle modification is an important component of treatment of hypertension. These measures should be initiated in patients with prehypertension (BP 120–140 systolic mm Hg), and continued even after starting antihypertensive drug therapy.

While it is commonly perceived that these are difficult to implement, it is important that the physician and other health care providers regularly reinforce these habits. Interventions should be tailored to an individual's cultural beliefs and with the support of their family. Simultaneously targeting multiple factors that impede BP control will maximize the likelihood of success [32]. Maintaining a normal BMI by reduction in calorie intake and regular physical activity is important not only for reduction in blood pressure, but for overall cardiovascular risk reduction. The DASH diet which emphasizes fruits and vegetables has been shown to lower blood pressure in African-American hypertensives [33]. Restriction of dietary sodium to 1,500 mg per day is particularly important in African Americans [34]. Alcohol intake should be limited (men: no more than 2 beers, 1 glass of wine, or 1 shot of whiskey (or hard liquor) per day and women: no more than 1 beer or 1 glass of wine per day [6]). Smoking cessation is an important adjunct in management of hypertension.

Drug Therapy in African Americans with Hypertension

As in most patients with hypertension, choice of antihypertensive drug therapy in African Americans is guided by the presence of coexistent medical conditions. For example, the presence of proteinuria favors initiation of inhibitors of the renin–angiotensin axis, and beta blockers are a rational choice in patients with hypertension and coronary artery disease. It is also important to appreciate that many patients will require more than one antihypertensive drug to achieve and maintain blood pressure control. Therefore, JNC-7 and the ISHIB guidelines recommend that in patients whose blood pressure is >15/10 mmHg above target, treatment can be initiated with a combination of two drugs [18, 19].

In patients with blood pressure ≤10 mmHg above target levels, and no compelling indications for a particular class, monotherapy with a diuretic or calcium channel blocker is reasonable.

Thiazide diuretics are effective in lowering blood pressure in African-American patients [35]. In addition, diuretics are unsurpassed by other antihypertensive drug classes in preventing long-term cardiovascular complications of hypertension in blacks [36]. While most clinical trials have used chlorthalidone, hydrochlorothiazide is the most commonly used thiazide diuretic in clinical practice. Chlorthalidone is more potent in lowering blood pressure and has a longer duration of action than hydrochlorothiazide [37]. Metabolic complications such hypokalemia are common with thiazide diuretics and require periodic lab monitoring. Thiazides are also more commonly associated with new onset diabetes than other antihypertensive drug therapy, though the clinical significance of this is uncertain [38].

Calcium channel blockers, particularly dihydropyridines, are effective in lowering blood pressure in African-American patients [39]. In the ALLHAT study, amlodipine was as effective as thiazide diuretic in preventing most long-term cardiovascular outcomes with the exception of heart failure [40]. In patients with chronic kidney disease and proteinuria, amlodipine was less effective than ramipril in preventing kidney disease outcomes; therefore, ACE inhibitor is preferred over calcium channel blockers as initial therapy in this setting [41]. Finally, the non-hydropyridine calcium channel blockers such as diltiazem and verapamil, while effective in lowering blood pressure, can lower heart rate, and should be used with caution when other negative chronotropic agents.

ACEI inhibitors as first line therapy are less effective than other classes of agents on lowering blood pressure in African-American hypertensives [42]. However, his difference is ameliorated with the addition of diuretic therapy [42]. In African-American patients with chronic kidney disease, ACE-based therapy is preferred over beta blockers and calcium channel blockers [41]. Angioedema is a rare, but serious side effect of ACE inhibitor therapy; it is more common in African Americans than other racial ethnic groups [43].

The use of nonselective betablockers as first line therapy in hypertension is generally no longer encouraged in the absence of a compelling indication; beta blockers have been shown to be less effective than other antihypertensive drugs in reducing cardiovascular morbidity and mortality [44]. This may relate to lack of reduction of central blood pressure with beta blocker-based treatment [45].

Other classes of antihypertensive agents such as vasodilators, centrally acting agents, and alpha blockers can be used in African-American patients if frontline drugs are not tolerated or additional antihypertensive drug therapy is required. Hydralazine in combination with nitrates is particularly effective in African-American patients with congestive heart failure [46]. Spironolactone is also a useful addition in patients with resistant hypertension.

In patients whose blood pressure is >15/10 mmHg above target, treatment can be initiated with a combination of two drugs. The ISHIB guidelines recommend the use of a RAS inhibitor and calcium channel blocker combination; however, use of the RAS inhibitor and diuretic combination may also be reasonable, particularly in patients with clinical evidence of volume overload.

Patients in whom blood pressure remains elevated despite optimal doses of three medications are considered to have resistant hypertension [47]. A systematic evaluation of blood pressure measurement, adherence, and use of medications that may be interfering with blood pressure control, optimizing antihypertensive drug therapy often results in improved blood pressure control. In these patients additional evaluation for secondary hypertension should also be considered.

In conclusion, hypertension is common, often poorly controlled, and contributes to premature morbidity and mortality in African-American patients. A careful clinical evaluation, appropriate use of lifestyle modifications, and rational choice of antihypertensive drug therapy can result in improved care and outcomes in this high-risk population.

References

1. http://www.cdc.gov/bloodpressure/facts.htm. 2011.
2. Carson AP, Howard G, Burke GL, Shea S, Levitan EB, Muntner P. Ethnic differences in hypertension incidence among middle-aged and older adults: the multi-ethnic study of atherosclerosis. Hypertension. 2011;57:1101–7.

3. Ford ES. Trends in mortality from all causes and cardiovascular disease among hypertensive and nonhypertensive adults in the United States. Circulation. 2011;123:1737–44.
4. Redmond N, Baer HJ, Hicks LS. Health behaviors and racial disparity in blood pressure control in the national health and nutrition examination survey. Hypertension. 2011;57:383–9.
5. Ogden CL, Carroll MD, Curtin LR, McDowell MA, Tabak CJ, Flegal KM. Prevalence of overweight and obesity in the United States, 1999–2004. JAMA. 2006;295:1549–55.
6. Flack JM, Sica DA, Bakris G, Brown AL, Ferdinand KC, Grimm Jr RH, et al. Management of high blood pressure in Blacks: an update of the International Society on Hypertension in Blacks consensus statement. Hypertension. 2010;56:780–800.
7. Peters RM, Flack JM. Salt sensitivity and hypertension in African Americans: implications for cardiovascular nurses. Prog Cardiovasc Nurs. 2000;15:138–44.
8. Calhoun DA. Hypertension in blacks: socioeconomic stress and sympathetic nervous system activity. Am J Med Sci. 1992;304:306–11.
9. Heffernan KS, Jae SY, Wilund KR, Woods JA, Fernhall B. Racial differences in central blood pressure and vascular function in young men. Am J Physiol Heart Circ Physiol. 2008;295:H2380–7.
10. Wang J, Chen W, Ruan L, Toprak A, Srinivasan SR, Berenson GS. Differential effect of elevated blood pressure on left ventricular geometry types in black and white young adults in a community (from the Bogalusa Heart Study). Am J Cardiol. 2011;107:717–22.
11. Okin PM, Kjeldsen SE, Dahlof B, Devereux RB. Racial differences in incident heart failure during antihypertensive therapy. Circ Cardiovasc Qual Outcomes. 2011;4:157–64.
12. Collins AJ, Foley RN, Herzog C, Chavers B, Gilbertson D, Ishani A, et al. US renal data system 2010 annual data report. Am J Kidney Dis. 2011;57:A8, e1-526.
13. Genovese G, Friedman DJ, Ross MD, Lecordier L, Uzureau P, Freedman BI, et al. Association of trypanolytic ApoL1 variants with kidney disease in African Americans. Science. 2010;329:841–5.
14. Liebson PR. Cardiovascular disease in special populations III: stroke. Prev Cardiol. 2010;13:1–7.
15. Pickering TG, Hall JE, Appel LJ, Falkner BE, Graves J, Hill MN, et al. Recommendations for blood pressure measurement in humans and experimental animals: part 1: blood pressure measurement in humans: a statement for professionals from the Subcommittee of Professional and Public Education of the American Heart Association Council on High Blood Pressure Research. Circulation. 2005;111:697–716.
16. Pickering TG, White WB. ASH position paper: home and ambulatory blood pressure monitoring. When and how to use self (home) and ambulatory blood pressure monitoring. J Clin Hypertens (Greenwich). 2008;10:850–5.
17. Pogue V, Rahman M, Lipkowitz M, Toto R, Miller E, Faulkner M, et al. Disparate estimates of hypertension control from ambulatory and clinic blood pressure measurements in hypertensive kidney disease. Hypertension. 2009;53:20–7.
18. Chobanian AV, Bakris GL, Black HR, Cushman WC, Green LA, Izzo Jr JL, et al. The seventh report of the Joint National Committee on prevention, detection, evaluation, and treatment of high blood pressure: the JNC 7 report. JAMA. 2003;289:2560–72.
19. Cushman WC, Evans GW, Byington RP, Goff Jr DC, Grimm Jr RH, Cutler JA, et al. Effects of intensive blood-pressure control in type 2 diabetes mellitus. N Engl J Med. 2010;362: 1575–85.
20. Appel LJ, Wright Jr JT, Greene T, Agodoa LY, Astor BC, Bakris GL, et al. Intensive blood-pressure control in hypertensive chronic kidney disease. N Engl J Med. 2010;363:918–29.
21. Wright Jr JT, Agodoa LY, Appel L, Cushman WC, Taylor AL, Obegdegbe GG, et al. New recommendations for treating hypertension in black patients: evidence and/or consensus? Hypertension. 2010;56:801–3.
22. Cushman WC, Ford CE, Cutler JA, Margolis KL, Davis BR, Grimm RH, et al. Success and predictors of blood pressure control in diverse North American settings: the antihypertensive and lipid-lowering treatment to prevent heart attack trial (ALLHAT). J Clin Hypertens (Greenwich). 2002;4:393–404.

23. Wright Jr JT, Agodoa L, Contreras G, Greene T, Douglas JG, Lash J, et al. Successful blood pressure control in the African American Study of kidney disease and hypertension. Arch Intern Med. 2002;162:1636–43.
24. Bosworth HB, Olsen MK, Grubber JM, Powers BJ, Oddone EZ. Racial differences in two self-management hypertension interventions. Am J Med. 2011;124:468.
25. Brennan T, Spettell C, Villagra V, Ofili E, McMahill-Walraven C, Lowy EJ, et al. Disease management to promote blood pressure control among African Americans. Popul Health Manag. 2010;13:65–72.
26. Houston TK, Allison JJ, Sussman M, Horn W, Holt CL, Trobaugh J, et al. Culturally appropriate storytelling to improve blood pressure: a randomized trial. Ann Intern Med. 2011;154: 77–84.
27. Victor RG, Ravenell JE, Freeman A, Leonard D, Bhat DG, Shafiq M, et al. Effectiveness of a barber-based intervention for improving hypertension control in black men: the BARBER-1 study: a cluster randomized trial. Arch Intern Med. 2011;171:342–50.
28. Einhorn PT. National heart, lung, and blood institute-initiated program "interventions to improve hypertension control rates in African Americans": background and implementation. Circ Cardiovasc Qual Outcomes. 2009;2:236–40.
29. Manze M, Rose AJ, Orner MB, Berlowitz DR, Kressin NR. Understanding racial disparities in treatment intensification for hypertension management. J Gen Intern Med. 2010;25:819–25.
30. Bell CN, Thorpe Jr RJ, Laveist TA. Race/Ethnicity and hypertension: the role of social support. Am J Hypertens. 2010;23:534–40.
31. Kressin NR, Orner MB, Manze M, Glickman ME, Berlowitz D. Understanding contributors to racial disparities in blood pressure control. Circ Cardiovasc Qual Outcomes. 2010;3:173–80.
32. Scisney-Matlock M, Bosworth HB, Giger JN, Strickland OL, Harrison RV, Coverson D, et al. Strategies for implementing and sustaining therapeutic lifestyle changes as part of hypertension management in African Americans. Postgrad Med. 2009;121:147–59.
33. Svetkey LP, Erlinger TP, Vollmer WM, Feldstein A, Cooper LS, Appel LJ, et al. Effect of lifestyle modifications on blood pressure by race, sex, hypertension status, and age. J Hum Hypertens. 2005;19:21–31.
34. Appel LJ, Giles TD, Black HR, Izzo Jr JL, Materson BJ, Oparil S, et al. ASH position paper: dietary approaches to lower blood pressure. J Am Soc Hypertens. 2010;4:79–89.
35. Materson BJ, Reda DJ, Cushman WC, Massie BM, Freis ED, Kochar MS, et al. Single-drug therapy for hypertension in men. A comparison of six antihypertensive agents with placebo. The department of veterans affairs cooperative study group on antihypertensive agents. N Engl J Med. 1993;328:914–21.
36. Wright Jr JT, Dunn JK, Cutler JA, Davis BR, Cushman WC, Ford CE, et al. Outcomes in hypertensive black and nonblack patients treated with chlorthalidone, amlodipine, and lisinopril. JAMA. 2005;293:1595–608.
37. Ernst ME, Carter BL, Goerdt CJ, Steffensmeier JJ, Phillips BB, Zimmerman MB, et al. Comparative antihypertensive effects of hydrochlorothiazide and chlorthalidone on ambulatory and office blood pressure. Hypertension. 2006;47:352–8.
38. Barzilay JI, Davis BR, Cutler JA, Pressel SL, Whelton PK, Basile J, et al. Fasting glucose levels and incident diabetes mellitus in older nondiabetic adults randomized to receive 3 different classes of antihypertensive treatment: a report from the Antihypertensive and Lipid-Lowering Treatment to Prevent Heart Attack Trial (ALLHAT). Arch Intern Med. 2006;166:2191–201.
39. Sareli P, Radevski IV, Valtchanova ZP, Libhaber E, Candy GP, Den Hond E, et al. Efficacy of different drug classes used to initiate antihypertensive treatment in black subjects: results of a randomized trial in Johannesburg. S Afr Arch Intern Med. 2001;161:965–71.
40. ALLHAT Officers and Coordinators for the ALLHAT Collaborative Research Group. The Antihypertensive and Lipid-Lowering Treatment to Prevent Heart Attack Trial. Major outcomes in high-risk hypertensive patients randomized to angiotensin-converting enzyme inhibitor or calcium channel blocker vs diuretic: the Antihypertensive and Lipid-Lowering Treatment to Prevent Heart Attack Trial (ALLHAT). JAMA. 2002;288:2981–97.

41. Wright Jr JT, Bakris G, Greene T, Agodoa LY, Appel LJ, Charleston J, et al. Effect of blood pressure lowering and antihypertensive drug class on progression of hypertensive kidney disease: results from the AASK trial. JAMA. 2002;288:2421–31.
42. Saunders E, Gavin JR. Blockade of the renin-angiotensin system in African Americans with hypertension and cardiovascular disease. J Clin Hypertens (Greenwich). 2003;5:12–7.
43. Piller LB, Ford CE, Davis BR, Nwachuku C, Black HR, Oparil S, et al. Incidence and predictors of angioedema in elderly hypertensive patients at high risk for cardiovascular disease: a report from the Antihypertensive and Lipid-Lowering Treatment to Prevent Heart Attack Trial (ALLHAT). J Clin Hypertens (Greenwich). 2006;8:649–56.
44. Lavie CJ, Messerli FH, Milani RV. Beta-blockers as first-line antihypertensive therapy the crumbling continues. J Am Coll Cardiol. 2009;54:1162–4.
45. Kamran H, Salciccioli L, Bastien C, Castro P, Sharma A, Lazar JM. Effect of beta blockers on central aortic pressure in African-Americans. J Am Soc Hypertens. 2011;5:94–101.
46. Taylor AL, Ziesche S, Yancy CW, Carson P, Ferdinand K, Taylor M, et al. Early and sustained benefit on event-free survival and heart failure hospitalization from fixed-dose combination of isosorbide dinitrate/hydralazine: consistency across subgroups in the African-American heart failure trial. Circulation. 2007;115:1747–53.
47. Calhoun DA, Jones D, Textor S, Goff DC, Murphy TP, Toto RD, et al. Resistant hypertension: diagnosis, evaluation, and treatment: a scientific statement from the American Heart Association Professional Education Committee of the Council for High Blood Pressure Research. Circulation. 2008;117:e510–26.

Chapter 4
Hypertension in Chronic Kidney Disease

Kunal Chaudhary, J.P. Buddineni, Joshua Botdorf,
and Adam Whaley-Connell

Introduction

The role of chronic elevations in blood pressure in the development of CKD is well recognized but underappreciated among clinicians. Clinically, both hypertension and kidney disease per se are relatively asymptomatic and thereby individuals and clinicians alike are unaware making this a complex relationship to detect. It has been well noted that hypertension is a cardiovascular risk factor that contribute to the development of chronic kidney disease (CKD). Hypertension is noted in approximately 61–66% of those with estimated glomerular filtration rate (eGFR) of <60 mL/min/1.73 m² [1]. As eGFR diminishes over time, the prevalence of hypertension increases with 36% in stage 1 CKD to 84% in stages 4–5 CKD [1]. Moreover, the prevalence of CKD in patients diagnosed with HTN is 27.5% compared to 22% among those with undiagnosed HTN [2]. It is also of worth noting that mortality from high blood pressure is more than double in low to middle income countries when compared to high income countries. As per 2009 global world health report, only 7% of deaths are caused due to high blood pressure in high income countries compared to 25% in African countries, for population under age 60 years [3].

K. Chaudhary, M.D. (✉) • A. Whaley-Connell
Division of Nephrology and Hypertension, Harry S. Truman VA Medical Center,
800 Hospital Dr, Columbia, MO 65211, USA

Department of Internal Medicine, University of Missouri-Columbia School
of Medicine, Columbia, MO, USA
e-mail: chaudharyk@health.missouri.edu

J.P. Buddineni • J. Botdorf
Department of Internal Medicine, University of Missouri-Columbia School
of Medicine, Columbia, MO, USA
e-mail: buddinenij@health.missouri.edu

S.I. McFarlane and G.L. Bakris (eds.), *Diabetes and Hypertension: Evaluation and Management*, Contemporary Diabetes, DOI 10.1007/978-1-60327-357-2_4,
© Springer Science+Business Media New York 2012

The Role of Hypertension in Cardiovascular Mortality in CKD

Approximately 13% of the US population has CKD [4]. Furthermore, the presence of CKD is associated with a high burden of cardiovascular disease (CVD) [5–8]. Mortality from CVD is approximately 10–30 times higher in CKD patients undergoing dialysis than in the general population [9]. Moreover, recent studies support that even early stages of CKD pose a significant risk factor of CVD [10]. The notion then that many patients with CKD may not even survive to require dialysis has many investigators interested in alternative strategies to detect and intervene in earlier stages of CKD [11]. The reverse relationship between CKD and CVD also holds true. Approximately 25% of patients with coronary artery disease, 33% of patients with acute myocardial infarction, and 50% of patients with heart failure have an eGFR less than 60 mL/min/1.73 m^2 [10, 12, 13]. Findings from the Atherosclerotic Risk in Communities (ARIC) suggest that CVD is an independent risk factor for development of kidney disease [14]. The excessive CVD risk burden in kidney disease has prompted the National Kidney Foundation (NKF) task force to consider CKD as a coronary artery disease equivalent for purposes of risk stratification [15].

Hypertension Goals in CKD Patients

There have been several studies reporting the beneficial effects of treating hypertension in patients with CKD by reducing proteinuria and slowing the decline in GFR and progression of CKD disease per se [16–18]. However, recent epidemiological studies have demonstrated the reverse paradigm that a lower blood pressure may be associated with a higher mortality in the ESRD patient population [19–23]. Several randomized controlled studies have tested the use of various antihypertensive groups of medications such as beta-blockers [24], angiotensin-converting enzyme inhibitors [25], and calcium channel blockers [26]. However, it is generally thought most of these trails are of smaller scale and may lack power to truly establish benefits of antihypertensive therapy in this unique population. A few meta-analyses studies suggest the beneficial effect of antihypertensive therapy in reducing CVD events in ESRD; however, no firm targets have been proposed to which blood pressure should be lowered to in such patients [27, 28]. Moreover, the presence of masked and white coat hypertension has been reported in the ESRD population confounding which measure to use in management of hypertension [29]. Aggressive treatment of hypertension in ESRD based only on blood pressure recordings either in the clinic or during dialysis sessions may lead to organ hypoperfusion. Few recent studies using home blood pressure monitoring in ESRD patients achieved better blood pressure target ranges [30, 31]. Unfortunately, there have been no out-of-dialysis unit blood pressure monitoring randomized control trials to better understand the lowering of blood pressure in high-risk populations.

Until large-scale randomized control trials both in and out of dialysis units are conducted, use of collective existing evidence suggests that high blood pressure should be treated among hypertensive individuals in CKD/ESRD population. It is still open for debate to the extent of blood pressure control in these high-risk populations. Due to lack of studies, it is also difficult to ascertain whether normotensive CKD patients would benefit from antihypertensive therapy.

Etiology/Pathophysiology

Volume-dependent hypertension. One major factor responsible for elevations in blood pressure in more advanced stages of CKD is expansion of extracellular fluid volume (ECF). Expansion of the ECF compartment is consistent with impaired natriuretic response in CKD population, after loading with sodium [32]. It has further been noted that there are greater increases in plasma volume compared to the ECF volume in subjects with CKD than without when isotonic saline is administered [33].

Dietary sodium intake. In the context of volume expansion, the significance of dietary sodium in maintenance of ECF volume has been well documented for many years [34, 35]. Dietary ingestion of sodium has shown to have a dose-dependent relationship with elevations in blood pressure. Modest reductions of sodium intake to 100 mmol per day have been shown to significantly reduce both systolic and diastolic blood pressure in both hypertensive and normotensive subjects in as little as 4 weeks [36]. Epidemiological studies further support a direct correlation between blood pressure and sodium intake; a meta-analysis of randomized control studies done by Midgley et al. has clearly demonstrated that sodium restriction would lead to decrease in blood pressure readings [37]. Moreover, modest dietary sodium restriction has been shown to improve long-term cardiovascular outcomes in general population [38, 39].

Renin–angiotensin system (RAS). Inappropriate activation of the RAS in the setting of adequate salt intake and volume expansion with elevations in angiotensin II (Ang II) has been well studied as a pro-inflammatory cytokine/pro-oxidant that contributes to kidney tissue injury [40]. This peptide fragment activates circulatory cells, causes endothelial damage, and facilitates the adhesion of molecules to the endothelial surface thus promoting inflammation via reactive oxygen species (ROS) production and nuclear factor kappa-B [41], subsequently potentiating hypertension-induced tissue damage [42, 43]. Furthermore, Ang II has also been noted to promote cell growth and fibrosis [44]. Thus, the pharmacological blockade of RAS is beneficial not only in reducing blood pressure, but also result in putative renoprotective effects.

Sympathetic nervous system (SNS). Inappropriate activation of sympathetic nervous system has been a well-studied concept leading to hypertension in CKD along with sodium retention and an altered pressure natriuresis relationship [45]. A significant role of neural mechanisms in CKD leading to hypertension was first suggested by McGrath et al., wherein subjects with CKD received autonomic blockade with atropine, prazosine, and propranolol and demonstrated a decrease in blood pressure not explained by volume overload and Ang II [46]. Following this seminal observation, many studies reinforced the role of sympathetic activation as a major role player contributing to hypertension in CKD [47, 48].

Secondary hyperparathyroidism. The development of elevations in parathyroid hormone levels is a common complication as a result of decreased renal function, vitamin D deficiency along with impaired mineral metabolism [49]. Secondary hyperparathyroidism in CKD is associated with several complications including renal osteodystrophy, extraskeletal calcification, and CVD as evidenced by left ventricular hypertrophy, vascular calcification, and congestive heart failure [50]. Despite the lack of large-scale randomized control study in defining the link between secondary hyperparathyroidism and CVD risk, observational data support a strong association between CVD mortality, parathyroid hormone, serum phosphate, and calcium product levels [51]. A retrospective study conducted by Goto et al. noted that parathyroidectomy in CKD patients with advanced secondary hyperparathyroidism led to improvement in left ventricular ejection fraction [52].

Erythropoietin associated factors. There has been ever expanding clinical use of recombinant erythropoietin in the past two decades from initial use in severely anemic hemodialysis patients to predialysis patients and a few subgroups of oncology patients. Two randomized controlled studies (CHOIR and CREATE) published in 2006 in predialysis patients suggest that use of recombinant erythropoietin was associated with higher cardiovascular adverse event rates and significant increases in hypertension [53, 54]. Even though there are no controlled intervention studies to elucidate the mechanisms of erythropoietin causing hypertension, the putative mechanisms include hypersensitivity to Ang II and norepinephrine [55, 56] as well as increased endothelin-1 [57, 58] activity in ESRD patient populations.

Management

The treatment of hypertension in those with CKD includes both nonpharmacologic and pharmacologic approaches. Current guidelines based on JNC-7 advocate for a blood pressure goal in those with CKD at <130/80 mmHg [59, 60]. This goal is supported by several studies suggesting a lower blood pressure may slow CKD progression. A meta-analysis in 2003 reported a lowered risk of CKD progression with a goal blood pressure of 110–129 mmHg and an increase in the relative risk for CKD progression at blood pressures above 130 mmHg. The beneficial results were most notable in patients with proteinuria exceeding 1 g per day [61].

Lifestyle and Dietary Approaches

The evidence for nonpharmacologic intervention for hypertension is compelling in the general population and has been largely extrapolated to the CKD population in clinical practice. Importantly, compliance and patient preferences are the biggest challenges for instituting lifestyle changes, and they should be a component of all successful pharmacologic regimens. Lifestyle modifications recommended by Kidney Disease Outcomes Quality Initiative (KDOQI) and the Canadian Society of Nephrology include smoking cessation, weight reduction, exercise, and restricting dietary sodium intake [60, 62].

Low Sodium Diet

Dietary sodium restriction is recommended to reduce extracellular fluid volume expansion and lower blood pressure. Sodium intake has a dose-dependent relationship with blood pressure, and a modest reduction of 55 mmol per day significantly reduced systolic and diastolic blood pressure as well as proteinuria in hypertensive subjects in as little as 4 weeks [63]. Blood pressure reduction with salt restriction can be seen across nondiabetic hypertensive ethnic groups, including Blacks, Hispanics, and Asians. Reduced sodium intake can lessen the incidence of hypertension by approximately 20% [64]. Excess sodium intake leads to resistance to renin–angiotensin–aldosterone system (RAAS) blockade and sodium restriction can be as effective as the addition of a thiazide to a therapeutic regimen containing angiotensin-converting enzyme (ACE) inhibitors or angiotensin II receptor blockers (ARB) [65, 66].

Weight Loss

Obesity is an independent risk factor for development and progression of CKD [67]. Reductions in body mass index (BMI) in obese patients with CKD with nonsurgical interventions can markedly decrease systolic blood pressure and proteinuria, along with cessation of GFR loss. Surgical intervention in morbidly obese individuals with a BMI >40 kg/m^2 has the potential for normalization of GFR and reduction of systolic blood pressure and micro-albuminuria [68]. The K/DOQI extends the JNC-7 recommendations for weight loss to a level of BMI <25 for those overweight and CKD to maintenance of weight of those with a BMI <25 [59, 60]. Avoidance of high protein diets is advised in light of the exorbitant amounts of protein in the Western diet and potential risk for enhancement of progression of CKD. Conversely, very restrictive diets may put the CKD patients at risk for malnutrition as these patients are already prone to protein-energy malnutrition which has been found be a predictor for mortality in these patients. Thereby, current thought is to promote a healthy lifestyle with modest protein intake.

As in general population, physical activity may provide a benefit. Although physical activity and the relationship have not been well studied in the CKD population, there appears to be a survival benefit in the CKD/ESRD population that participates in regular physical activity [69].

Pharmacologic Interventions

Diuretics

Diuretics along with salt restriction have become a cornerstone for the treatment of hypertension in association with CKD. While salt is effective in the early stages of CKD, diuretics become essential when sodium restriction alone is unsatisfactory in CKD [70]. Thiazides can cause a 10–15 and 5–10 mmHg reduction in the systolic and diastolic blood pressures, respectively [71]. Besides volume depletion, decreases in systemic vascular resistance accounts for the antihypertensive effects of thiazide diuretics. However, thiazide diuretics lose much of their antihypertensive effects when GFR falls below 45 ml/min/1.73 m^2 and are generally effective with an eGFR of >30 ml/min/1.73 m^2 [60]. Hydrochlorothiazide (HCTZ) is the most widely used thiazide used for treating high blood pressure; chlorthalidone maybe more efficacious in reducing blood pressure [72–75]. In a major clinical trial Chlorthalidone was shown to be as effective as CCBs and ACEI in prevention of cardiovascular disease as well as less expensive [75]. Some side effects of thiazide diuretics include hyperglycemia, hyperuricemia, hypercalcemia, and hypokalemia and hypomagnesemia, which are dose dependent.

As the GFR declines, loop diuretics are needed for effective volume management. Loop diuretics for volume control and hypertension work in two stages, initiation and maintenance. Once the patient has achieved a maximum diuresis without symptoms of orthostatic hypotension, cramps, fatigue, or decreased renal function, then the patient should be titrated down to the lowest dose necessary to maintain established dry weight [76]. As CKD worsens and the dose needs to be monitored and adjusted to maintain dry weight, increased doses of loop diuretics are required with diminishing kidney function and inadequately dosed furosemide administration will result in sodium retention. Due to its short acting nature furosemide should be dosed at least twice daily. Other loop diuretics such as Bumetanide and Torsemide have better bioavailability as compared to Furosemide; however, clinically the effects are the same when dosed equivalently. Prolonged use of loop diuretics often leads to diuretic resistance due to hypertrophy of distal tubular cells, which can be overcome by adding a Thiazide such as Metolazone, which works on the distal tubules.

Inhibition of the Renin–Angiotensin–Aldosterone System (RAAS)

RAAS inhibition is considered as first line therapy by both the K/DOQI and the JNC [7, 59, 60] and most commonly with angiotensin converting enzyme (ACE) inhibitors and angiotensin II receptor blockers (ARB). ACE inhibitors competitively block the action of ACE, thereby reducing circulating levels of angiotensin II (Ang II) whereas ARBs specifically block the binding of Ang II to the angiotensin type I receptor (AT1R). Blockage of RAAS system offsets direct vasoconstriction, release of noradrenaline from sympathetic nerve terminals, stimulation of proximal tubular reabsorption of sodium, stimulation of aldosterone secretion, and vasopressin release, which not only reduces blood pressure in the CKD patient but also reduces the progression of CKD in nondiabetic kidney disease and proteinuria [77–79]. Like the ACE inhibitors, ARBs also reduce blood pressure, decrease proteinuria, and limit CKD progression in diabetic kidney disease [80, 81], and possibly nondiabetic kidney disease as well [82]. The utility of combination ARB-ACE inhibition also display greater reductions in proteinuria than monotherapy; however, these comparisons are at conventional doses and monotherapy at higher doses may be of equal benefit [82, 83]. A major limitation with the use of ACE inhibitor and ARB regimens in the CKD population is the risk for hyperkalemia and the odds of mortality increase when hyperkalemia is present [84]. The risk of hyperkalemia can be mitigated by the concomitant use of diuretics [85], dietary potassium restriction, and potassium resin binders.

Mineralocorticoid receptor (MR) antagonists offer an additional RAAS blockage in those with resistant hypertension. Their role is also limited due to potential risk for hyperkalemia in those with advanced CKD. Spironolactone and eplerenone are the MR antagonists that potentially prevent the aldosterone escape mechanism that occurs with ACE inhibitors and ARB [86]. There is significant reduction in blood pressure and proteinuria when these MR antagonists are added to an ACE inhibitor or ARB [87, 88]. The beneficial cardiac results in patients with CVD have been shown, but have not been duplicated in patients with an eGFR <60 ml/min/1.73 m^2 [89]. Adverse effects associated with MR antagonists include breast tenderness, gynecomastia, hyperkalemia, prostatic hypertrophy, erectile dysfunction, and menstrual irregularities. Eplerenone is generally better tolerated with reduced anti-androgenic side effects and gynecomastia, but needs to be used with caution with inhibitors of CYP3A4 such as Verapamil and Diltiazem. The incidence of hyperkalemia (>5.5 mmol/l) is approximately 5.7 % in those with an eGFR <60 ml/min/1.73 m^2 and greater in those with an eGFR <45 ml/min/1.73 m^2 [90].

Direct renin inhibition has become available and some evidence supports its use in CKD patients. In patients with type 2 diabetes mellitus, hypertension, and diabetic kidney disease, combination therapy with maximal doses of losartan and aliskiren had a 20 % reduction in albuminuria as compared to losartan and placebo [91]. Serum potassium elevations >5.5 mmol/l were more frequent with aliskiren (22.5 %) versus placebo (13.6 %) in stage 3 CKD [92]. All other adverse event rates were similar between treatments, irrespective of CKD stage, except for an increased rate of renal dysfunction seen in the aliskiren group in stage 3 CKD patients [92].

As additional studies and comparisons to other RAAS agent are performed, the role of aliskiren in clinical practice will be better understood. At this time aliskiren is recommended to patients that have incomplete RAAS blockade with an eGFR >30 ml/min/1.73 m². Additionally, when evaluated in type 2 diabetic patients with albuminuria, the combination is more antiproteinuric than monotherarpy with ARB. Aliskiren is contraindicated for use with ARBs or ACEIs in patients with diabetes because of the risk of renal impairment, hypotension, and hyperkalemia. A warning to avoid use of aliskiren with ARBs or ACEIs in patients with moderate to severe renal impairment (i.e., where glomerular filtration rate [GFR] <60 ml/min) has been issued

Calcium Channel Blockers

Calcium channel blockers can be used as second-line antihypertensive agents and are a good alternative for patients who have side effects to ACE inhibitors and ARBs. They are effective at reducing CKD progression and cardiovascular events when used in combination with other agents [75]. The non-dihydropuridines subclass besides lowering blood pressure, also decreases glomerular pressure and reduce proteinuria. However the dihydropuridine subclass reduces blood pressure but have no change on glomerular pressure and are inconsistent with the degree of reduction in proteinuria [93]. Both the classes of calcium channel blockers in proteinuric nephropathies reduce proteinuria when used along with an ACE inhibitor or an ARB. They have been shown to preserve renal function in both diabetics and nondiabetics with proteinuria [78, 91]. When verapamil and ramipril are combined, the level of protein reduction is nearly double when dosed for similar blood pressure reductions [93]. Thus CCBs can be used either as monotherapy or to complement existing antihypertensive therapy in CKD hypertensive patients.

β-Blockers

Sympathetic overactivity in CKD contributes to the maintenance of hypertension, thus β blockers have a theoretical benefit in the treatment of hypertension in those with CKD. In the African American Study of Kidney Disease (AASK), metoprolol was not as effective as ACE inhibtors in slowing GFR decline. However, metoprolol did have a reduced risk of ESRD and mortality benefit in as compared to amlodipine [94]. This data is strong evidence in support of using cardioselective β-blockers in CKD. Vasodilating β-blockers, labetalol, and carvedilol have been used in hypertensive patients with renal impairment. While blood pressure reduction can be achieved, data is limited with the use of labetalol with regard to CKD progression and proteinuria [95]. Studies with carvedilol indicate that renal blood flow and GFR are preserved with reductions in micro-albuminuria in both diabetic and nondiabetic hypertensives with micro-albuminuria [96]. Carvedilol has a significant mortality benefit in ESRD patients with heart failure, but large prospective trials evaluating the use in CKD are lacking. Nevibilol, a newer agent with vasodilatory properties, has proven to be safe in those with CKD stage 3 [97]. In animals the agent has shown to provide reductions in proteinuria and renal fibrosis [98]. Caution should be exercised with certain β-blockers such as Atenolol, which can accumulate in CKD patients and cause side effects without additional BP control. Clearly β-blockers play an important role in those with cardiovascular disease and CKD, but it is not a first line agent and should be reserved for those with other compelling indications.

Endothelin Antagonism

Endothelin has been implicated in CKD progression and podocyte injury, and intervention may be beneficial. Two agents so far have been evaluated for use in hypertension, avosentan, and darusentan [99]. The addition of avosentan in CKD stage 3 and 4 patients with diabetic nephropathy as a complementary agent results in a significant reduction in proteinuria independent of decreased blood pressure. These findings have also been duplicated in nondiabetic CKD as well [100, 101]. AZ significant adverse reaction is sodium and fluid retention that may lead to congestive heart failure, the ASCEND trial was prematurely ended for this reason. Additional studies evaluating CKD progression, mortality, and cardiovascular outcomes are needed before the role of endothelin antagonists are established.

α-Blockers

α-blockers are generally not considered as first line therapy, but may have a role in resistant hypertension by blocking vasoconstricting α-1 adrenoreceptors on vascular smooth muscles. Combination of doxazosin, was effective in combining with ACE inhibitors, calcium channel blockers, β-blockers, and diuretics in nondiabetic CKD patients in the Anglo-Scandinavian Cardiac Outcomes Trial–Blood Pressure Lowering Arm (ASCOT–BPLA) whose blood pressure remains above 140/90 mmHg. There was no apparent excess of heart failure among doxazosin users in that study and plasma lipid profiles were improved [102]. However, when compared to chlorthalidone in ALLHAT, doxazosin had higher risks of heart failure with similar rates of stroke and combined cardiovascular disease [103]. The decision to employee α-1 antagonists should balance these increased risks. Other adverse events include nasal congestion and dizziness. α-blockers do cause sodium retention causing expansion of plasma volume, which can be more evident in CKD patients, and diuretic therapy may be needed, which may exacerbate the orthostatic hypotension seen with these drugs.

Central Sympatholytic

Clonidine, which is typically administered orally or as a transdermal patch is the most commonly used central sympatholytic, successfully reduces blood pressure and has neutral effects upon proteinuria. Clonidine stimulates both a2-adrenergic receptors and I1-imidazoline receptors in the rostral ventrolateral medulla nuclei resulting in decreased sympathetic outflow. Transdermal patches have several advantages that include continuous drug delivery, improved compliance, decreased rebound upon stopping, and decreased side effects that include somnolence and dry mouth [104]. Due to prolongation of half-life in CKD patients, the rebound effect is somewhat lower than is otherwise expected. Skin reactions are common with the transdermal patch. Sodium retention can occur with central sympatholytics and diuretics may be required. CKD patients with sinus node dysfunction can be at risk for significant bradycardia and its use specially in combination with beta blockers in such patients should be avoided.

Vasodilators

Direct vasodilators, i.e., hydralazine and minoxidil, are available for blood pressure control. Both are considered 4th line agents and only used when hypertensive goals have not been reached with other agents. Although being used for many years, the effects of the agent on mortality, morbidity, and renal outcomes are poorly understood [105]. A common side effect reflexive tachycardia can be controlled with β-blockers or a centrally acting α-agonist. When combined with a nitrate significant reduction in mortality in blacks with heart failure was seen, but this has not been specifically studied in the setting of CKD [106].

Minoxidil, is an adjunctive therapy in cases poorly responsive, severe hypertension in CKD. Hypertension, even in the setting in of CKD, is at least partially responsive to minoxidil. Minoxidil, while more efficacious in the degree of blood pressure reduction compared to hydralazine, has a more significant side effect profile [107]. Simultaneous administration of a diuretic with a β-blocker or a combined α–β blocker is often required to control edema and tachycardia associated with minoxidil use. Sodium retention due to minoxidil can be the cause of significant edema or pericardial effusion often resulting in temporary cessation of the medication. A loop diuretic or the addition of metolazone is required in some cases [108].

References

1. U.S. Renal Data System, USRDS 2010 Annual Data Report: Atlas of Chronic Kidney Disease and End-Stage Renal Disease in the United States, National Institutes of Health, National Institute of Diabetes and Digestive and Kidney Diseases, Bethesda, MD, 2010.
2. Crews DC, Plantinga LC, Miller ER 3rd, Saran R, Hedgeman E, Saydah SH, et al. Prevalence of chronic kidney disease in persons with undiagnosed or prehypertension in the United States. Hypertension. 2010;55(5): 1102–9.

3. 2009 WHO Global Health report. Available at: http://www.who.int/healthinfo/global_burden_disease/en/index.html.
4. Coresh J, Selvin E, Stevens LA, et al. Prevalence of chronic kidney disease in the United States. JAMA. 2007;298(17):2038–47.
5. Berl T, Henrich W. Kidney-heart interactions: epidemiology, pathogenesis, and treatment. Clin J Am Soc Nephrol. 2006;1(1):8–18.
6. Coca SG, Krumholz HM, Garg AX, Parikh CR. Underrepresentation of renal disease in randomized controlled trials of cardiovascular disease. JAMA. 2006;296(11):1377–84.
7. Garg AX, Clark WF, Haynes RB, House AA. Moderate renal insufficiency and the risk of cardiovascular mortality: results from the NHANES I. Kidney Int. 2002;61(4):1486–94.
8. Go AS, Chertow GM, Fan D, McCulloch CE, Hsu CY. Chronic kidney disease and the risks of death, cardiovascular events, and hospitalization. N Engl J Med. 2004;351(13): 1296–305.
9. Sarnak MJ, Levey AS, Schoolwerth AC, Coresh J, Culleton B, Hamm LL, et al. Kidney disease as a risk factor for development of cardiovascular disease: a statement from the American Heart Association Councils on Kidney in Cardiovascular Disease, High Blood Pressure Research, Clinical Cardiology, and Epidemiology and Prevention. Circulation. 2003;108(17):2154–69.
10. Anavekar NS, McMurray JJ, Velazquez EJ, Solomon SD, Kober L, Rouleau JL, et al. Relation between renal dysfunction and cardiovascular outcomes after myocardial infarction. N Engl J Med. 2004;351(13):1285–95.
11. Keith DS, Nichols GA, Gullion CM, Brown JB, Smith DH. Longitudinal follow-up and outcomes among a population with chronic kidney disease in a large managed care organization. Arch Intern Med. 2004;164(6):659–63.
12. Shlipak MG, Smith GL, Rathore SS, Massie BM, Krumholz HM. Renal function, digoxin therapy, and heart failure outcomes: evidence from the digoxin intervention group trial. J Am Soc Nephrol. 2004;15(8):2195–203.
13. Ix JH, Shlipak MG, Liu HH, Schiller NB, Whooley MA. Association between renal insufficiency and inducible ischemia in patients with coronary artery disease: the heart and soul study. J Am Soc Nephrol. 2003;14(12):3233–8.
14. Elsayed EF, Tighiouart H, Griffith J, et al. Cardiovascular disease and subsequent kidney disease. Arch Intern Med. 2007;167(11):1130–6.
15. Levey AS, Beto JA, Coronado BE, et al. Controlling the epidemic of cardiovascular disease in chronic renal disease: what do we know? What do we need to learn? Where do we go from here? National Kidney Foundation Task Force on Cardiovascular Disease. Am J Kidney Dis. 1998;32(5):853–906.
16. Jafar TH, Stark PC, Schmid CH, Landa M, Maschio G, de Jong PE, et al. Progression of chronic kidney disease: the role of blood pressure control, proteinuria, and angiotensin-converting enzyme inhibition: a patient-level meta-analysis. Ann Intern Med. 2003;139(4): 244–52.
17. Sarnak MJ, Greene T, Wang X, Beck G, Kusek JW, Collins AJ et al. The effect of a lower target blood pressure on the progression of kidney disease: long-term follow-up of the modification of diet in renal disease study. Ann Intern Med. 2005;142(5):342–51.
18. Wright JT Jr, Bakris G, Greene T, Agodoa LY, Appel LJ, Charleston J, et al. Effect of blood pressure lowering and antihypertensive drug class on progression of hypertensive kidney disease: results from the AASK trial. JAMA. 2002;288(19):2421–31.
19. Kalantar-Zadeh K, Kilpatrick RD, McAllister CJ, Greenland S, Kopple JD. Reverse epidemiology of hypertension and cardiovascular death in the hemodialysis population: the 58th annual fall conference and scientific sessions. Hypertension. 2005;45(4):811–7.
20. Port FK, Hulbert-Shearon TE, Wolfe RA, et al. Predialysis blood pressure and mortality risk in a national sample of maintenance hemodialysis patients. Am J Kidney Dis. 1999;33(3):507–17.
21. Zager PG, Nikolic J, Brown RH, Campbell MA, Hunt WC, Peterson D, et al. "U" curve association of blood pressure and mortality in hemodialysis patients. Medical Directors of Dialysis Clinic, Inc. Kidney Int. 1998;54(2):561–9.

22. Li Z, Lacson E Jr, Lowrie EG, Ofsthun NJ, Kuhlmann MK, Lazarus JM, et al. The epidemiology of systolic blood pressure and death risk in hemodialysis patients. Am J Kidney Dis. 2006;48(4):606–15.
23. Agarwal R. Hypertension in chronic kidney disease and dialysis: pathophysiology and management. Cardiol Clin. 2005;23(3):237–48.
24. Cice G, Ferrara L, D'Andrea A, D'Isa S, Di Benedetto A, Cittadini A, et al. Carvedilol increases two-year survivalin dialysis patients with dilated cardiomyopathy: a prospective, placebo-controlled trial. J Am Coll Cardiol. 2003;41(9):1438–44.
25. Zannad F, Kessler M, Lehert P, et al. Prevention of cardiovascular events in end-stage renal disease: results of a randomized trial of fosinopril and implications for future studies. Kidney Int. 2006;70(7):1318–24.
26. Tepel M, Hopfenmueller W, Scholze A, Maier A, Zidek W. Effect of amlodipine on cardiovascular events in hypertensive haemodialysis patients. Nephrol Dial Transplant. 2008;23(11):3605–12.
27. Heerspink HJ, Ninomiya T, Zoungas S, et al. Effect of lowering blood pressure on cardiovascular events and mortality in patients on dialysis: a systematic review and meta-analysis of randomised controlled trials. Lancet. 2009;373(9668):1009–15.
28. Agarwal R, Sinha AD. Cardiovascular protection with antihypertensive drugs in dialysis patients: systematic review and meta-analysis. Hypertension. 2009;53(5):860–6.
29. Bangash F, Agarwal R. Masked hypertension and white-coat hypertension in chronic kidney disease: a meta-analysis. Clin J Am Soc Nephrol. 2009;4(3):656–64.
30. Cappuccio FP, Kerry SM, Forbes L, Donald A. Blood pressure control by home monitoring: meta-analysis of randomised trials. BMJ. 2004;329(7458):145.
31. Alborzi P, Patel N, Agarwal R. Home blood pressures are of greater prognostic value than hemodialysis unit recordings. Clin J Am Soc Nephrol. 2007;2(6):1228–34.
32. Koomans HA, Roos JC, Dorhout Mees EJ, Delawi IM. Sodium balance in renal failure. A comparison of patients with normal subjects under extremes of sodium intake. Hypertension. 1985;7(5):714–21.
33. Koomans HA, Geers AB, Boer P, Roos JC, Dorhout Mees EJ. A study on the distribution of body fluids after rapid saline expansion in normal subjects and in patients with renal insufficiency: preferential intravascular deposition in renal failure. Clin Sci (Lond). 1983;64(2):153–60.
34. Murphy RJ. The effect of "rice diet" on plasma volume and extracellular fluid space in hypertensive subjects. J Clin Invest. 1950;29(7):912–7.
35. Watkin DM, Froeb HG, Hatch FT, Gutman AB. Effects of diet in essential hypertension. II. Results with unmodified Kempner rice diet in 50 hospitalized patients. Am J Med. 1950;9(4):441–93.
36. He FJ, Marciniak M, Visagie E, et al. Effect of modest salt reduction on blood pressure, urinary albumin, and pulse wave velocity in white, black, and Asian mild hypertensives. Hypertension. 2009;54(3):482–8.
37. Midgley JP, Matthew AG, Greenwood CM, Logan AG. Effect of reduced dietary sodium on blood pressure: a meta-analysis of randomized controlled trials. JAMA. 1996;275(20):1590–7.
38. Cook NR, Cutler JA, Obarzanek E, Buring JE, Rexrode KM, Kumanyika SK, et al. Long term effects of dietary sodium reduction on cardiovascular disease outcomes: observational follow-up of the trials of hypertension prevention (TOHP). BMJ. 2007;334(7599):885–8.
39. Weinberger MH, Fineberg NS. Sodium and volume sensitivity of blood pressure. Age and pressure change over time. Hypertension. 1991;18(1):67–71.
40. Ruiz-Ortega M, Esteban V, Rupérez M, Sánchez-López E, Rodríguez-Vita J, Carvajal G, et al. Renal and vascular hypertension-induced inflammation: role of angiotensin II. Curr Opin Nephrol Hypertens. 2006;15(2):159–66.
41. Esteban V, Lorenzo O, Ruperez M, et al. Angiotensin II, via AT1 and AT2 receptors and NF-kappaB pathway, regulates the inflammatory response in unilateral ureteral obstruction. J Am Soc Nephrol. 2004;15(6):1514–29.

42. Suzuki Y, Ruiz-Ortega M, Lorenzo O, Ruperez M, Esteban V, Egido J. Inflammation and angiotensin II. Int J Biochem Cell Biol. 2003;35(6):881–900.
43. Endemann DH, Schiffrin EL. Endothelial dysfunction. J Am Soc Nephrol. 2004;15(8): 1983–92.
44. Ruiz-Ortega M, Ruperez M, Esteban V, Egido J. Molecular mechanisms of angiotensin II-induced vascular injury. Curr Hypertens Rep. 2003;5(1):73–9.
45. Orth SR, Amann K, Strojek K, Ritz E. Sympathetic overactivity and arterial hypertension in renal failure. Nephrol Dial Transplant. 2001;16 Suppl 1:67–9.
46. McGrath BP, Tiller DJ, Bune A, Chalmers JP, Korner PI, Uther JB. Autonomic blockade and the Valsalva maneuver in patients on maintenance hemodialysis: a hemodynamic study. Kidney Int. 1977;12(4):294–302.
47. Converse Jr RL, Jacobsen TN, Toto RD, et al. Sympathetic overactivity in patients with chronic renal failure. N Engl J Med. 1992;327(27):1912–8.
48. Campese VM, Kogosov E. Renal afferent denervation prevents hypertension in rats with chronic renal failure. Hypertension. 1995;25(4 Pt 2):878–82.
49. Coladonato JA, Ritz E. Secondary hyperparathyroidism and its therapy as a cardiovascular risk factor among end-stage renal disease patients. Adv Ren Replace Ther. 2002;9(3):193–9.
50. Joy MS, Karagiannis PC, Peyerl FW. Outcomes of secondary hyperparathyroidism in chronic kidney disease and the direct costs of treatment. J Manag Care Pharm. 2007;13(5):397–411.
51. Levin NW, Hoenich NA. Consequences of hyperphosphatemia and elevated levels of the calcium-phosphorus product in dialysis patients. Curr Opin Nephrol Hypertens. 2001;10(5):563–8.
52. Goto N, Tominaga Y, Matsuoka S, Sato T, Katayama A, Haba T, et al. Cardiovascular complications caused by advanced secondary hyperparathyroidism in chronic dialysis patients; special focus on dilated cardiomyopathy. Clin Exp Nephrol. 2005;9(2):138–41.
53. Singh AK, Szczech L, Tang KL, et al. Correction of anemia with epoetin alfa in chronic kidney disease. N Engl J Med. 2006;355(20):2085–98.
54. Drüeke TB, Locatelli F, Clyne N, Eckardt KU, Macdougall IC, Tsakiris D, et al. Normalization of hemoglobin level in patients with chronic kidney disease and anemia. N Engl J Med. 2006;355(20):2071–84.
55. Hand MF, Haynes WG, Johnstone HA, Anderton JL, Webb DJ. Erythropoietin enhances vascular responsiveness to norepinephrine in renal failure. Kidney Int. 1995;48(3):806–13.
56. Yamakado M, Umezu M, Nagano M, Tagawa H. Mechanisms of hypertension induced by erythropoietin in patients on hemodialysis. Clin Invest Med. 1991;14(6):623–9.
57. Takahashi K, Totsune K, Imai Y, et al. Plasma concentrations of immunoreactive-endothelin in patients with chronic renal failure treated with recombinant human erythropoietin. Clin Sci (Lond). 1993;84(1):47–50.
58. Kang DH, Yoon KI, Han DS. Acute effects of recombinant human erythropoietin on plasma levels of proendothelin-1 and endothelin-1 in haemodialysis patients. Nephrol Dial Transplant. 1998;13(11):2877–83.
59. Chobanian AV, Bakris GL, Black HR, Cushman WC, Green LA, Izzo JL Jr, Jones DW, Materson BJ, Oparil S, Wright JT Jr, Roccella EJ; National Heart, Lung, and Blood Institute Joint National Committee on Prevention, Detection, Evaluation, and Treatment of High Blood Pressure; National High Blood Pressure Education Program Coordinating Committee. The Seventh Report of the Joint National Committee on Prevention, Detection, Evaluation, and Treatment of High Blood Pressure: the JNC 7 report. JAMA. 2003;289(19):2560–72.
60. Kidney Disease Outcomes Quality Initiative (K/DOQI). K/DOQI clinical practice guidelines on hypertension and antihypertensive agents in chronic kidney disease. Am J Kidney Dis. 2004;43(5 suppl 2):S1–290.
61. Jafar TH, Stark PC, Schmid CH, Landa M, Maschio G, de Jong PE, et al. Progression of chronic kidney disease: the role of blood pressure control, proteinuria, and angiotensin-converting enzyme inhibition: a patient-level metaanalysis. Ann Intern Med. 2003;139(4):244–52.
62. Levin A, Hemmelgarn B, Culleton B, Tobe S, McFarlane P, Ruzicka M, Canadian Society of Nephrology, et al. Guidelines for the management of chronic kidney disease. CMAJ. 2008;179(11):1154–62.

63. He FJ, Marciniak M, Visagie E, Markandu ND, Anand V, Dalton RN, et al. Effect of modest salt reduction on blood pressure, urinary albumin, and pulse wave velocity in white, black, and Asian mild hypertensives. Hypertension. 2009;54(3):482–8.

64. Effects of weight loss and sodium reduction intervention on blood pressure and hypertension incidence in overweight people with high normal blood pressure: the Trials of Hypertension Prevention, phase II: the Trials of Hypertension Prevention Collaborative Research Group. Arch Intern Med. 1997;157:657–667.

65. Buter H, Hemmelder MH, Navis G, de Jong PE, de Zeeuw D. The blunting of the antiproteinuric efficacy of ACE inhibition by high sodium intake can be restored by hydrochlorothiazide. Nephrol Dial Transplant. 1998;13(7):1682–5.

66. Vogt L, Waanders F, Boomsma F, de Zeeuw D, Navis G. Effects of dietary sodium and hydrochlorothiazide on the antiproteinuric efficacy of losartan. J Am Soc Nephrol. 2008;19(5):999–1007.

67. Wang Y, Chen X, Song Y, Caballero B, Cheskin LJ. Association between obesity and kidney disease: A systematic review and meta-analysis. Kidney Int. 2008;73:19–33.

68. Navaneethan SD, Yehnert H, Moustarah F, Schreiber MJ, Schauer PR, Beddhu S. Weight loss interventions in chronic kidney disease: a systematic review and meta-analysis. Clin J Am Soc Nephrol. 2009;4(10):1565–74.

69. Beddhu S, Baird BC, Zitterkoph J, Neilson J, Greene T. Physical activity and mortality in chronic kidney disease (NHANES III). Clin J Am Soc Nephrol. 2009;4(12):1901–6.

70. Buter H, Hemmelder MH, Navis G, de Jong PE, de Zeeuw D. The blunting of the antiproteinuric efficacy of ACE inhibition by high sodium intake can be restored by hydrochlorothiazide. Nephrol Dial Transplant. 1998;13(7):1682–5.

71. Ernst ME, Moser M. Use of diuretics in patients with hypertension. N Engl J Med. 2009;361(22):2153–64.

72. Rahman M, Pressel S, Davis BR, Nwachuku C, Wright Jr JT, Whelton PK, et al. Renal outcomes in high-risk hypertensive patients treated with an angiotensin-converting enzyme inhibitor or a calcium channel blocker vs a diuretic: a report from the Antihypertensive and Lipid-Lowering Treatment to Prevent Heart Attack Trial (ALLHAT). Arch Intern Med. 2005;165(8):936–46.

73. Multiple Risk Factor Intervention Trial Research Group. Multiple risk factor intervention trial: risk factor changes and mortality results. JAMA. 1982;248:1465–77.

74. Ernst ME, Carter BL, Goerdt CJ, Steffensmeier JJ, Phillips BB, Zimmerman MB, et al. Comparative antihypertensive effects of hydrochlorothiazide and chlorthalidone on ambulatory and office blood pressure. Hypertension. 2006;47(3):352–8.

75. ALLHAT Officers and Coordinators for the ALLHAT Collaborative Research Group. The Antihypertensive and Lipid-Lowering Treatment to Prevent Heart Attack Trial. Major outcomes in high-risk hypertensive patients randomized to angiotensin-converting enzyme inhibitor or calcium channel blocker vs. diuretic: The Antihypertensive and Lipid-Lowering Treatment to Prevent Heart Attack Trial (ALLHAT). JAMA. 2002;88:2981–97.

76. Zamboli P, De Nicola L, Minutolo R, Bertino V, Catapano F, Conte G. Management of hypertension in chronic kidney disease. Curr Hypertens Rep. 2006;8(6):497–501.

77. Jafar TH, Schmid CH, Landa M, Giatras I, Toto R, Remuzzi G, et al. Angiotensin-converting enzyme inhibitors and progression of nondiabetic renal disease. A meta-analysis of patient-level data. Ann Intern Med. 2001;135(2):73–87.

78. The GISEN. Group (Gruppo Italiano di Studi Epidemiologici in Nefrologia). Randomized placebo-controlled trial of effect of ramipril on decline in glomerular filtration rate and risk of terminal renal failure in proteinuric, non-diabetic nephropathy. Lancet. 1997;349:1857–63.

79. Barnett AH, Bain SC, Bouter P, Karlberg B, Madsbad S, Jervell J, et al. Diabetics Exposed to Telmisartan and Enalapril Study Group. Angiotensin-receptor blockade versus converting-enzyme inhibition in type 2 diabetes and nephropathy. N Engl J Med. 2004;351(19):1952–61.

80. Brenner BM, Cooper ME, de Zeeuw D, Keane WF, Mitch WE, Parving HH, et al. Effects of losartan on renal and cardiovascular outcomes in patients with type 2 diabetes and nephropathy. N Engl J Med. 2001;345(12): 861–9.
81. Lewis EJ, Hunsicker LG, Clarke WR, et al. Renoprotective effect of the angiotensin receptor antagonist irbesartan in patients with nephropathy due to type 2 diabetes. N Engl J Med. 2001;345(12):851–60.
82. Li PK, Leung CB, Chow KM, Cheng YL, Fung SK, Mak SK, et al. HKVIN Study Group. Hong Kong study using valsartan in IgA nephropathy (HKVIN): a double-blind, randomized, placebo-controlled study. Am J Kidney Dis. 2006;47(5):751–60.
83. Kunz R, Friedrich C, Wolbers M, Mann JF. Meta-analysis: effect of monotherapy and combination therapy with inhibitors of the renin angiotensin system on proteinuria in renal disease. Ann Intern Med. 2008;148(1):30–48.
84. Einhorn LM, Zhan M, Hsu VD, Walker LD, Moen MF, Seliger SL, et al. The frequency of hyperkalemia and its significance in chronic kidney disease. Arch Intern Med. 2009;169(12):1156–62.
85. Weinberg JM, Appel LJ, Bakris G, Gassman JJ, Greene T, Kendrick CA, et al. African American Study of Hypertension and Kidney Disease Collaborative Research Group. Risk of hyperkalemia in nondiabetic patients with chronic kidney disease receiving antihypertensive therapy. Arch Intern Med. 2009;169(17):1587–94.
86. Bomback AS, Klemmer PJ. The incidence and implications of aldosterone breakthrough. Nat Clin Pract Nephrol. 2007;3(9):486–92.
87. Bomback AS, Kshirsagar AV, Amamoo MA, Klemmer PJ. Change in proteinuria after adding aldosterone blockers to ACE inhibitors or angiotensin receptor blockers in CKD: a systematic review. Am J Kidney Dis. 2008;51(2):199–211.
88. Navaneethan SD, Nigwekar SU, Sehgal AR, Strippoli GF. Aldosterone antagonists for preventing the progression of chronic kidney disease: a systematic review and meta-analysis. Clin J Am Soc Nephrol. 2009;4(3):542–51.
89. Pitt B, Zannad F, Remme WJ, Cody R, Castaigne A, Perez A, et al. The effect of spironolactone on morbidity and mortality in patients with severe heart failure. Randomized Aldactone Evaluation Study Investigators. N Engl J Med. 1999;341(10):709–17.
90. Heshka J, Ruzicka M, Hiremath S, McCormick BB. Spironolactone for difficult to control hypertension in chronic kidney disease: an analysis of safety and efficacy. J Am Soc Hypertens. 2010;4(6):295–301.
91. Parving HH, Persson F, Lewis JB, Lewis EJ, Hollenberg NK. AVOID Study Investigators. Aliskiren combined with losartan in type 2 diabetes and nephropathy. N Engl J Med. 2008;358(23):2433–46.
92. Persson F, Lewis JB, Lewis EJ, Rossing P, Hollenberg NK, Parving HH. AVOID Study Investigators. Impact of baseline renal function on the efficacy and safety of aliskiren added to losartan in patients with type 2 diabetes and nephropathy. Diabetes Care. 2010;33(11):2304–9.
93. Toto RD. Management of hypertensive chronic kidney disease: role of calcium channel blockers. J Clin Hypertens (Greenwich). 2005;7(4 Suppl 1):15–20.
94. Wright Jr JT, Bakris G, Greene T, Agodoa LY, Appel LJ, Charleston J, et al. Effect of blood pressure lowering and antihypertensive drug class on progression of hypertensive kidney disease: results from the AASK trial. JAMA. 2002;288(19):2421–31.
95. Bakris GL, Hart P, Ritz E. Beta blockers in the management of chronic kidney disease. Kidney Int. 2006;70(11):1905–13.
96. Bakris GL, Fonseca V, Katholi RE, et al. Metabolic effects of carvedilol vs metoprolol in patients with type 2 diabetes mellitus and hypertension: a randomized controlled trial. JAMA. 2004;292:2227–36.
97. Cohen-Solal A, Kotecha D, van Veldhuisen DJ, Babalis D, Böhm M, Coats AJ, et al. Efficacy and safety of nebivolol in elderly heart failure patients with impaired renal function: insights from the SENIORS trial. Eur J Heart Fail. 2009;11(9):872–80.

98. Whaley-Connell A, Habibi J, Johnson M, Tilmon R, Rehmer N, Rehmer J, et al. Nebivolol reduces proteinuria and renal NADPH oxidase-generated reactive oxygen species in the transgenic Ren2 rat. Am J Nephrol. 2009;30(4):354–60.
99. Moore R, Linas S. Endothelin antagonists and resistant hypertension in chronic kidney disease. Curr Opin Nephrol Hypertens. 2010;19(5):432–6.
100. Dhaun N, MacIntyre IM, Melville V, et al. Blood pressure-independent reduction in proteinuria and arterial stiffness after acute endothelin: a receptor antagonism in chronic kidney disease. Hypertension. 2009;54:113–9.
101. Mann JF, Green D, Jamerson K, Ruilope LM, Kuranoff SJ, Littke T, et al. ASCEND Study Group. Avosentan for overt diabetic nephropathy. J Am Soc Nephrol. 2010;21(3):527–35.
102. Mori Y, Matsubara H, Nose A, Shibasaki Y, Masaki H, Kosaki A, et al. Safety and availability of doxazosin in treating hypertensive patients with chronic renal failure. Hypertens Res. 2001;24(4):359–63.
103. Davis BR, Cutler JA, Furberg CD, ALLHAT Collaborative Research Group, et al. Relationship of antihypertensive treatment regimens and change in blood pressure to risk for heart failure in hypertensive patients randomly assigned to doxazosin or chlorthalidone: further analyses from the Antihypertensive and Lipid-Lowering treatment to prevent Heart Attack Trial. Ann Intern Med. 2002;137:313–20.
104. Mancia G, Parati G, Pomodosi G, et al. Evaluation of the antihypertensive effects of TTS clonidine by multiple 24-hr automatic Blood pressure monitoring. J Cardiovasc Pharmacol. 1987;10(S12):S187–93.
105. Kandler MR, Mah GT, Tejani AM, Stabler SN. Hydralazine for essential hypertension. Cochrane Database Syst Rev. 2010;(8):CD004934.
106. Taylor AL, Ziesche S, Yancy C, Carson P, D'Agostino Jr R, Ferdinand K, et al. Combination of isosorbide dinitrate and hydralazine in blacks with heart failure. N Engl J Med. 2004;351(20):2049–57.
107. Gottlieb TB, Katz FH, Chidsey 3rd CA. Combined therapy with vasodilator drugs and beta-adrenergic blockade in hypertension. A comparative study of minoxidil and hydralazine. Circulation. 1972;45(3):571–82.
108. Sica DA. Minoxidil: an underused vasodilator for resistant or severe hypertension. J Clin Hypertens (Greenwich). 2004;6(5):283–7.

Chapter 5
Diabetes and Hypertension in People with Sleep Apnea: Risk Evaluation and Therapeutic Rationale

Abhishek Pandey, Oladipupo Olafiranye, Monsur Adedayo, Ferdinand Zizi, Samy I. McFarlane, and Girardin Jean-Louis

Diabetes in People with Sleep Apnea: Risk Evaluation and Therapeutic Rationale

OSA: Definition and Epidemiology

Sleep apnea is a serious, potentially life-threatening condition, characterized by repeated cessation of breathing while sleeping. Sleep apnea is probably responsible for 38,000 cardiovascular deaths yearly, with an associated 42 million dollars spent on related hospitalizations [1]. Sleep apnea is a major public health problem, affecting an estimated 18 million Americans in the USA [2, 3]. Certain NIH reports have suggested sleep apnea to be as prevalent as adult diabetes [3–5]. Among middle-age adults, using a respiratory disturbance index ≥10, the Wisconsin Sleep Cohort Study estimated that sleep apnea affects as much as 24 % of men and 9 % of women [6]. Among an urban adult population in the Cleveland family study, 5 year incidence is 7.5–16 % for sleep disordered breathing, of which OSA is the most common type [7].

A. Pandey • M. Adedayo • F. Zizi • G. Jean-Louis, Ph.D. (✉)
Department of Medicine, Sleep Disorder and Disparity Centers,
SUNY Downstate Medical Center, Brooklyn, NY, USA
e-mail: girardin.jean-louis@downstate.edu

O. Olafiranye
Division of Cardiology, Department of Medicine,
SUNY Downstate Medical Center, Brooklyn, NY, USA

S.I. McFarlane, M.D., M.P.H., M.B.A.
Division of Endocrinology, Diabetes and Hypertension, Department of Medicine,
SUNY-Downstate and Kings County Hospital, Brooklyn, NY, USA
e-mail: Samy.McFarlane@downstate.edu

S.I. McFarlane and G.L. Bakris (eds.), *Diabetes and Hypertension: Evaluation and Management*, Contemporary Diabetes, DOI 10.1007/978-1-60327-357-2_5,
© Springer Science+Business Media New York 2012

Recent data strongly suggests that ethnicity should be considered as an important risk factor for OSA. A study among blacks in Brooklyn demonstrated that a history of CVD was the most important predictor expressing symptoms of sleep apnea, with an odds ratio of 11 [8]. Despite evidence that metabolic risk markers (e.g., obesity, HTN, and DM) for CVD are more prevalent among blacks [9], the vast majority of suspected cases in this population remain undiagnosed. This paints a population in which among the few that are screened, many are at risk for OSA or positive for OSA, suggesting substantial gains in diagnosis can be made by improving adherence. Underdiagnosis among blacks is of great concern since prevalence of OSA risk factors is higher in this population, an odds ratio of 1.88 when compared to whites [10].

Relationships Between Diabetes and Sleep Apnea

Prevalence of OSA in DM

Growing evidence has demonstrated pronounced relationship of sleep apnea on insulin resistance [11–14, 87–89]. Some estimates of prevalence of sleep apnea among diabetics as defined by the Sleep AHEAD (Action for Health in Diabetes) has been estimated to be as high as 86 % [15]. Data from the Sleep Heart Health Study indicated that patients with moderate sleep apnea (AHI≥ 15) had an increased risk of having impaired glucose tolerance [16]. Community data from the sleep laboratory at Queensberry hospital demonstrated each additional apneic event increased fasting insulin level by 0.5% [11]. Supporting evidence from the Nurse health study suggested that sleep loss induced by apnea is linked to worsening of type II diabetes [17]. The data showed that short sleepers (≤5 h per day) are more likely to be associated with diabetes. This is consistent with data from Quebec Family Study and Sleep Heart Health Study indicating that aberrant sleep durations (short sleep: ≤5 h and long sleep: ≥9 h) are associated with increased prevalence of diabetes and impaired glucose tolerance [18, 19]. According to data from the National Health and Nutrition Examination survey, it may be that individuals reporting fewer than 5 h of sleep or more than 9 h might be at increased risk of developing diabetes according to data from the National Health and Nutrition Examination survey [20].

Screening/Risk Evaluation

There is widespread lack of knowledge essential to make informed decisions about obtaining sleep assessment. Few people are aware of what constitutes a comprehensive sleep assessment. Few know the consequences of sleep apnea, ranging from annoying to life-threatening [12]. Sleep apnea is complex, requiring continued examination of at-risk individuals, who may not have the disease at one time, but who may subsequently develop it. Considering the health beliefs described above, it is possible that blacks in particular may not be aware that a disease such as OSA requires continuous screening.

Evidence from CPAP Studies

CPAP is the most effective, nonsurgical treatment for sleep apnea [21]. It consists of a patient fitted by a trained technician to wear a mask over the nose/mouth or both. The pressure in the oropharyngeal airway is titrated in a way to assess in maintaining airway patency. The standard of care according to the American Academy of Sleep Medicine [21] is usually accompanied by behavioral modification, especially to target the patient's body habitus. Combined treatment is catered to lessen physiological issues and risk from comorbidities as well as alleviate signs and symptoms.

Despite being effective in the management of sleep apnea, adherence to CPAP therapy remains a concern among healthcare providers. CPAP adherence is defined as the mean number of hours per day and days per week patients report using CPAP (adherence: >4 h for 70 % of the nights or no report of symptomatic complaints). Disappointing data indicates that more than half of the patients at the start of their treatment accepted CPAP devices [22]. Furthermore, a significant percentage of patients discontinued CPAP therapy during the first week [23, 24]. Factors that may increase CPAP adherence include satisfaction with management of the disease [25], adherence during the initial period [23], and personality characteristics [25, 26]. Educational programs that involve overcoming barriers in timely CPAP use, especially involving family members, have proven to be more successful [27]. These programs suggest improving lifestyle choices through weight reduction, increased physical activity, and tobacco avoidance [28, 29]. It is of critical importance that these intervention programs instituted in the first 2 weeks of treatment to remain and/or increase adherence a year later [28–33].

Investigations have demonstrated that continuous positive airway pressure (CPAP) studies produced significant improvement in glucose control and left ventricular function [34]. Evidence from clinical trials shows that CPAP therapy can also normalize leptin [35] and ghrelin [36] levels, thereby reducing central [37] and visceral obesity [38].

Studies have shown an overall beneficial effects among patients who adhered to standardized recommendations to use CPAP treatment (≥4 h per night) [27]. Certain interventional studies (Table 5.1) have shown that CPAP therapy can also be a crucial therapeutic modality in treatment of diabetic patients with sleep apnea. Harsch et al. [39] showed significant improvements in insulin sensitivity index (ISI), established by euglycaemic hyperinsulinaemic clamp tests, after 3 months of CPAP treatment. In a longitudinal trial of close to 3 years, German researchers indicated that regular and effective long-term CPAP treatment may improve insulin sensitivity [40]. Dawson et al. [41] demonstrated that sleeping glucose level was more stable after treatment, with the median SD decreasing from 20.0 to 13.0 mg/dL and the mean difference between maximum and minimum values decreasing from 88 to

Table 5.1 CPAP studies and reduction in glucose

Study/year	Response to therapy		Duration of CPAP usage in treatment arm
	Measurement of glucose metabolism	Change (posttreatment vs. baseline)	
Harsch [39]	Mean insulin sensitivity index (ISI)	4.38 ± 2.94 vs. 2.74 ± 2.25 μmol/kg × min	5.8 ± 1.2 h/night (3 months)
Babu [42]	Hemoglobin A$_{1c}$	8.6 % ± 1.8 % vs. 9.2 % ± 2.0 %	6.6 ± 2.0 h/night (83 ± 50 days)
Schahin et al. [40]	Mean insulin sensitivity Index (ISI)	10.6 ± 7.0 vs. 6.3 ± 5.6 μmol/kg × min	5.2 ± 1.6 h/night (2.9 years)
Dawson [41]	Mean sleeping glucose	102.9 ± 39.4 vs. 122.0 ± −61.7 mg/dL	Not reported (42 days)

57 mg/dL. Consistent with this finding, another adherence study showed that patients adhering to CPAP therapy had significantly reduced post-prandial glucose values and hemoglobin A$_{1C}$ level [42]. Another important finding from that study is that among patients who used CPAP for more than 4 h per day, the reduction in HBA$_{1C}$ level was correlated with days of CPAP use [42]. Adequate usage of CPAP therapy is effective in reducing global cardiovascular disease risk (18.8 ± 9.8 % vs. 13.9 ± 9.7 %, $p = 0.001$) [69]. Some randomized controlled trials found no statistically significant improvement therapeutic CPAP therapy on glucose metabolism [43]. Possible hypothesized mechanisms suggested by these investigators included severe insulin resistance and morbid obesity.

Therapeutic Rationale

We have shown through supportive evidence the associations between diabetes and sleep apnea.

These new findings are important, as they shed light into treatment approaches that rely only on pharmacotherapeutic management of diabetes, without consideration of possible overlying sleep apnea. Among diabetic patients, there is an inverse relationship between the severity of sleep apnea and glucose impairment, after controlling for multiple potential confounders, including obesity [34]. Moreover, compared to patients without sleep apnea, the presence of mild, moderate, or severe sleep apnea increased mean adjusted HbA$_{1c}$ values by 1.49, 1.93, and 3.69 %, respectively [34].

In light of current evidence, intense pharmacotherapy for diabetes should be coordinated with treatment for sleep apnea to reduce the cardiovascular burden. A comprehensive evaluation of sleep apnea and sleeping habits among patients with diabetes and other cardiometabolic risk profile patients seems warranted. Healthcare providers should consider non-pharmacological interventions (i.e., CPAP therapy), which might enhance effectiveness of traditional pharmacologic intervention and decrease unwanted pharmacological side effects.

Future Directions and Clinical Implications

Currently available data only sheds light to portions of this complex issue. The initial investigations regarding relationships between sleep apnea and the abnormal glucose metabolism have not addressed whether the impaired glucose metabolism represents a mediating factor in the link of sleep apnea to cardiovascular disease, or diabetes itself might potentiate the effects of sleep apnea on cardiovascular diseases. Studies testing causal models to explain links among these metabolic conditions and test cause-and-effect relationships of those factors are warranted.

Many interventions can be implemented to improve the management of existing metabolic disorders. First, as sleep apnea is highly prevalent among patients with diabetes, a sleep apnea screening questionnaire should be administered to those at-risk patients. Additionally, questionnaires should be administered to patients with increased visceral, abdominal, or neck adiposity. Second, patients at risk for sleep apnea should be referred to a sleep laboratory. Third, weight management programs should be designed to assist patients in their effort to reduce their body weight, as weight reduction helps diminish the severity of sleep apnea, thereby improving overall general health and quality of life. Fourth, patients on intensive pharmacotherapy for diabetes and worsening sleep apnea should avoid weight gain drugs whenever possible to prevent the worsening of sleep apnea and cardiovascular events.

It is evident that the recent rise in metabolic disorders such as obesity, diabetes, and sleep apnea is independent of age, gender, and geography. However, there is a greater public health concern about individuals living in at-risk, underserved communities that are traditionally underrepresented in the health care. African–Americans have a disproportionately higher prevalence of these conditions [44]. Thus, ultimately adequate management of sleep apnea among African Americans with sleep apnea will contribute to meaningful reductions of cardiovascular disease risk in this vulnerable population.

Hypertension in People with Sleep Apnea: Risk Evaluation and Therapeutic Rationale

Introduction

Hypertension is defined as blood pressure (BP) greater than 140/90 mmHg for the general adult population. Based on this BP cutoff for hypertension as defined by the seventh report of the Joint National Committee on Prevention, Detection, Evaluation, and Treatment of High Blood Pressure (JNC 7) [45], about 29 % of adult Americans, or approximately one-third of the American population, have hypertension [46]. OSA and Hypertension have more than a few characteristics in common. Both are common in obese middle-aged males, and both are often undiagnosed and associated with increased risk of cardiovascular damage. Above all, the striking epidemiology makes it most unlikely that this association is by chance. OSA is considered one of the secondary causes of hypertension in the Seventh Report of the Joint National Committee on Prevention, Detection, Evaluation, and Treatment of High Blood Pressure (JNC-7).

Hypertension affects approximately 50 % of people with OSA and conversely, approximately 40 % of hypertensive patients are diagnosed with OSA [47]. Based on the projections from the Wisconsin Sleep Cohort, OSA contributes to hypertension in 400,000 women and two million men in the USA [48]. These observations prompted the American Heart Association to issue a Scientific Statement describing the need to recognize OSA as an important target for therapy in reducing cardiovascular risk. Although several mechanisms have been suggested as possible linkage between hypertension and OSA, sustained adrenergic stimulation appears to be the most compelling pathophysiological link between the two. In this chapter we will discuss the pathophysiological and epidemiological data associating OSA with hypertension. Diagnosis and management of hypertension in OSA patients will also be discussed.

Pathophysiological Link Between OSA and Hypertension

The mechanisms by which OSA results in cardiovascular diseases and in particular hypertension is shown in Fig. 5.1 [49]. With upper airway obstruction, respiratory efforts against the collapsed glottis results in negative intrathoracic pressure and a decrease in stroke volume and BP [50]. This leads to activation of sympathetic nervous system via carotid chemoreceptors as a consequence of repetitive hypoxemia [51], increased carbon dioxide [52, 53], and decreased cardiac output [54]. The enhanced sympathetic activity results in increased vascular resistance and eventually an increase in cardiac output and BP. The repetitive hypoxemia have also been linked to generation of reactive oxygen species [55], vasoactive mediators [56], inflammatory markers [57], and activation of the renin–angiotensin–aldosterone–system (RAAS) [58], leading to fluid retention, endothelial dysfunction, and subsequent atherosclerosis. Observing this chain of events, investigators postulates that atherogenesis apparently starts soon after the onset of OSA and may constitute the mechanistic paradigm by which OSA mediates the genesis or worsening of hypertension [59].

Beyond the aforementioned, OSA also causes significant changes in intrathoracic pressure that increases transmural gradients across atria, ventricle, and aorta. This in turn disrupts the heart ventricular function as well as autonomic and hemodynamic stability [60–62]. The on toward effect may include increased afterload, thoracic aorta dilatation, and increased propensity for aortic dissection [63–66]. Also, the non-dipping phenomenon (attenuation of normal decrease in BP during sleep) [67] is often seen in patients with OSA and has been linked to increased all-cause mortality [68]. This increased nighttime BP has been suggested as a better prognostic factor for cardiovascular events [47, 68].

Fig. 5.1 The genesis of
hypertension and other
cardiovascular diseases in
obstructive sleep apnea.
Adapted from [86]

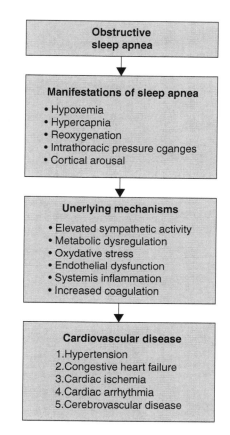

Patients with OSA have characteristically greater levels of endothelin and lower levels of nitric oxide than healthy sleepers [69, 70] This elevated endothelin concentration is believed to contribute to greater blood vessel constriction and peripheral vascular resistance and consequently hypertension. Notably, levels of endothelin and circulating nitric oxide invariably return to normal following treatment of OSA with CPAP [70]. Two large longitudinal studies, the Sleep Heart Health Study and the Wisconsin Sleep Cohort, showed higher risk of hypertension for individuals with higher OSA severity score [71, 72]. The Wisconsin Sleep Cohort Study demonstrated a consistent OSA-BP dose–response relationship, even after controlling for age, sex, BMI, and antihypertensive medications [72].

Management of Hypertension in Patients with OSA

Screening for OSA is very important in patients with hypertension. Approximately 85 % of adults with clinically significant and treatable OSA go undiagnosed [73]. Although obesity is the usual trigger for referral for evaluation of OSA, it has been suggested that OSA may be a stronger risk factor for hypertension in nonobese patients in comparison to obese patients [48, 74]. Thus, clinicians should not only consider habitus but should also be vigilant for symptoms of OSA using basic screening tools such as Epworth Sleepiness Scale to identify patients with symptoms of somnolence [30], the Berlin Questionnaire for OSA symptoms [75] and Apnea Risk Evaluation System (ARES) Questionnaire [76] to identify those at risk for OSA. In patients with suspected OSA, a definitive diagnosis often requires the gold standard for diagnosis of OSA—polysomnography that provides hemodynamic, encephalographic, and electrocardiographic data in addition to respiratory data [77].

Treatment of OSA involves risk factors modification and relieve of airway obstruction. CPAP therapy is usually considered as initial obstruction-relieving therapy in the management of hypertension in patients with OSA. This ventilation assist method transmits forced air into the oropharynx via a fitted mask over the nose (some methods use a mask fitted to both the nose and mouth) to help maintain a patent upper airway and reduce the effort of inhalation. Through the reduction of sympathetic activity, oxidative radicals, and inflammation [78], CPAP therapy results in lowering of BP. Three meta-analyses of randomized controlled trials summarized in a recent review estimated a statistically significant reduction in mean BP with the use of CPAP [47]. The meta-analysis with the greatest degree of BP reduction [79] estimated a mean reduction in systolic BP of 2.46 mmHg (95 % CI, 0.62–4.31 mmHg) and a mean reduction in diastolic BP of 1.83 mmHg (95 % CI, 0.61–3.05 mmHg). A smaller study of 11 similar patients demonstrated even more impressive findings in both systolic and diastolic BP with a decrease of 11.0±4.4 mmHg in 24-h systolic BP after 2 months of CPAP therapy. Nocturnal diastolic BP was reduced by 7.8±3.0 mmHg [80]. The duration of therapy and adherence to CPAP (>4 h for 70 % of the nights) appears to be important for a maximal therapeutic effect of CPAP therapy [50, 81].

Oral appliances and anatomical correction of upper airway by surgery have been used to prevent and/or relieve airway obstruction in OSA patient [82, 83]. However, their role in the treatment of hypertension remains controversial. The most common procedure is the revised uvulopalatopharyngoplasty for which a small study showed improvement in nighttime but not daytime BP [83].

If BP remains above goal despite optimal OSA treatment, antihypertensive therapy should be initiated or adjusted. Hypertension in patients with OSA is often resistant to treatment and a key element in management is to block RAAS with (ACE-I/ARB), decrease vasoconstriction with a vasodilator, and address volume overload with either a thiazide-type diuretic or a loop diuretic. In the absence of compelling indications, antihypertensive regimens should begin with a RAAS blocker (ACE-I/ARB), calcium channel blocker, or a diuretic [84] in different combination for optimal BP control [90]. Aldosterone antagonists have been found to be a potentially important adjunctive agent in the management of sleep apnea-induced hypertension given the relatively high prevalence of primary hyperaldosteronism [85, 86]. These agents induce added diuresis in combination with standard diuretics by reducing sodium reabsorption in the distal nephron.

Conclusion

Obstructive sleep apnea is a risk factor for hypertension. Optimal treatment of sleep apnea improves blood pressure control in hypertensive patients with sleep apnea.

References

1. Barthel SW, Strome M. Snoring, obstructive sleep apnea, and surgery. Med Clin North Am. 1999;83(1):85–96.
2. Gallup. 2000 Omnibus Sleep in America Poll. National Sleep Foundation 2000;1–19. Available at: URL: http://www.sleepfoundation.org/publications/2000poll.html. Accessed August 24, 2000.
3. Phillipson EA. Sleep apnea-a major public health problem. N Engl J Med. 1993;328(17): 1271–3.
4. Young T, Finn L. Epidemiological insights into the public health burden of sleep disordered breathing: sex differences in survival among sleep clinic patients. Thorax. 1998;53 Suppl 3: S16–9.
5. Omnibus Sleep in America Poll. National Sleep Foundation; 2005.
6. Young T, Palta M, Dempsey J, Skatrud J, Weber S, Badr S. The occurrence of sleep-disordered breathing among middle-aged adults. N Engl J Med. 1993;328(17):1230–5.
7. Tishler PV, Larkin EK, Schluchter MD, Redline S. Incidence of sleep-disordered breathing in an urban adult population: the relative importance of risk factors in the development of sleep-disordered breathing. J Am Med Assoc. 2003;289(17):2230–7.
8. Zizi F, Jean-Louis G, Fernandez S, et al. Symptoms of obstructive sleep apnea in a Caribbean sample. Sleep Breath. 2008;12(4):317–22.
9. Silverberg DS, Oksenberg A, Iaina A. Sleep-related breathing disorders as a major cause of essential hypertension: fact or fiction? Curr Opin Nephrol Hypertens. 1998;7(4):353–7.
10. Redline S, Tishler PV, Hans MG, Tosteson TD, Strohl KP, Spry K. Racial differences in sleep-disordered breathing in African-Americans and Caucasians. Am J Respir Crit Care Med. 1997;155(1):186–92.
11. Ip MS, Lam B, Ng MM, Lam WK, Tsang KW, Lam KS. Obstructive sleep apnea is independently associated with insulin resistance. Am J Respir Crit Care Med. 2002;165(5):670–6.
12. Punjabi NM, Sorkin JD, Katzel LI, Goldberg AP, Schwartz AR, Smith PL. Sleep-disordered breathing and insulin resistance in middle-aged and overweight men. Am J Respir Crit Care Med. 2002;165(5):677–82.
13. Punjabi NM, Shahar E, Redline S, Gottlieb DJ, Givelber R, Resnick HE. Sleep-disordered breathing, glucose intolerance, and insulin resistance: the Sleep Heart Health Study. Am J Epidemiol. 2004;160(6):521–30.
14. Punjabi NM, Polotsky VY. Disorders of glucose metabolism in sleep apnea. J Appl Physiol. 2005;99(5):1998–2007.
15. Foster GD, Sanders MH, Millman R, et al. Obstructive sleep apnea among obese patients with type 2 diabetes. Diabetes Care. 2009;32(6):1017–9.
16. Resnick HE, Redline S, Shahar E, et al. Diabetes and sleep disturbances: findings from the Sleep Heart Health Study. Diabetes Care. 2003;26(3):702–9.
17. Ayas NT, White DP, Al Delaimy WK, et al. A prospective study of self-reported sleep duration and incident diabetes in women. Diabetes Care. 2003;26(2):380–4.
18. Gottlieb DJ, Punjabi NM, Newman AB, et al. Association of sleep time with diabetes mellitus and impaired glucose tolerance. Arch Intern Med. 2005;165(8):863–7.
19. Tasali E, Leproult R, Spiegel K. Reduced sleep duration or quality: relationships with insulin resistance and type 2 diabetes. Prog Cardiovasc Dis. 2009;51(5):381–91.

20. Gangwisch JE, Heymsfield SB, Boden-Albala B, et al. Sleep duration as a risk factor for diabetes incidence in a large U.S. sample. Sleep. 2007;30(12):1667–73.
21. The American Academy of Sleep Medicine (Practice Parameters). http://www.aasmnet.org/practiceparameters.htm. Accessed August 24, 2002. Ref Type: Internet Communication
22. Wright J, Johns R, Watt I, Melville A, Sheldon T. Health effects of obstructive sleep apnoea and the effectiveness of continuous positive airways pressure: a systematic review of the research evidence. Br Med J. 1997;314(7084):851–60.
23. Rosenthal L, Gerhardstein R, Lumley A, et al. CPAP therapy in patients with mild OSA: implementation and treatment outcome. Sleep Med. 2000;1(3):215–20.
24. Anand VK, Ferguson PW, Schoen LS. Obstructive sleep apnea: a comparison of continuous positive airway pressure and surgical treatment. Otolaryngol Head Neck Surg. 1991;105(3):382–90.
25. Ball EM, Banks MB. Determinants of compliance with nasal continuous positive airway pressure treatment applied in a community setting. Sleep Med. 2001;2(3):195–205.
26. Fletcher EC, Shah A, Qian W, Miller III CC. "Near miss" death in obstructive sleep apnea: a critical care syndrome. Crit Care Med. 1991;19(9):1158–64.
27. Riley RW, Powell NB, Guilleminault C, Clerk A, Troell R. Obstructive sleep apnea. Trends in therapy. West J Med. 1995;162(2):143–8.
28. Hoy CJ, Vennelle M, Kingshott RN, Engleman HM, Douglas NJ. Can intensive support improve continuous positive airway pressure use in patients with the sleep apnea/hypopnea syndrome? Am J Respir Crit Care Med. 1999;159(4 Pt 1):1096–100.
29. Oki Y, Shiomi T, Sasanabe R, et al. Multiple cardiovascular risk factors in obstructive sleep apnea syndrome patients and an attempt at lifestyle modification using telemedicine-based education. Psychiatry Clin Neurosci. 1999;53(2):311–3.
30. Chervin RD, Theut S, Bassetti C, Aldrich MS. Compliance with nasal CPAP can be improved by simple interventions. Sleep. 1997;20(4):284–9.
31. Aloia MS, Di Dio L, Ilniczky N, Perlis ML, Greenblatt DW, Giles DE. Improving compliance with nasal CPAP and vigilance in older adults with OAHS. Sleep Breath. 2001;5(1):13–21.
32. Zozula R, Rosen R. Compliance with continuous positive airway pressure therapy: assessing and improving treatment outcomes. Curr Opin Pulm Med. 2001;7(6):391–8.
33. Popescu G, Latham M, Allgar V, Elliott MW. Continuous positive airway pressure for sleep apnoea/hypopnoea syndrome: usefulness of a 2 week trial to identify factors associated with long term use. Thorax. 2001;56(9):727–33.
34. Aronsohn RS, Whitmore H, Van CE, Tasali E. Impact of untreated obstructive sleep apnea on glucose control in type 2 diabetes. Am J Respir Crit Care Med. 2010;181(5):507–13.
35. Sanner BM, Kollhosser P, Buechner N, Zidek W, Tepel M. Influence of treatment on leptin levels in patients with obstructive sleep apnoea. Eur Respir J. 2004;23(4):601–4.
36. Takahashi K, Chin K, Akamizu T, et al. Acylated ghrelin level in patients with OSA before and after nasal CPAP treatment. Respirology. 2008;13(6):810–6.
37. Pillar G, Shehadeh N. Abdominal fat and sleep apnea: the chicken or the egg? Diabetes Care. 2008;31 Suppl 2:S303–9.
38. Trenell MI, Ward JA, Yee BJ, et al. Influence of constant positive airway pressure therapy on lipid storage, muscle metabolism and insulin action in obese patients with severe obstructive sleep apnoea syndrome. Diabetes Obes Metab. 2007;9(5):679–87.
39. Harsch IA, Schahin SP, Bruckner K, et al. The effect of continuous positive airway pressure treatment on insulin sensitivity in patients with obstructive sleep apnoea syndrome and type 2 diabetes. Respiration. 2004;71(3):252–9.
40. Schahin SP, Nechanitzky T, Dittel C, et al. Long-term improvement of insulin sensitivity during CPAP therapy in the obstructive sleep apnoea syndrome. Med Sci Monit. 2008;14(3):CR117–21.
41. Dawson A, Abel SL, Loving RT, et al. CPAP therapy of obstructive sleep apnea in type 2 diabetics improves glycemic control during sleep. J Clin Sleep Med. 2008;4(6):538–42.
42. Babu AR, Herdegen J, Fogelfeld L, Shott S, Mazzone T. Type 2 diabetes, glycemic control, and continuous positive airway pressure in obstructive sleep apnea. Arch Intern Med. 2005;165(4):447–52.

43. Clarenbach CF, West SD, Kohler M. Is obstructive sleep apnea a risk factor for diabetes? Discov Med. 2011;12(62):17–24.

44. Nunes J, Jean-Louis G, Zizi F, et al. Sleep duration among black and white Americans: results of the National Health Interview Survey. J Natl Med Assoc. 2008;100(3):317–22.

45. Chobanian AV, Bakris GL, Black HR, et al. The Seventh Report of the Joint National Committee on Prevention, Detection, Evaluation, and Treatment of High Blood Pressure: the JNC 7 report. J Am Med Assoc. 2003;289(19):2560–72.

46. Egan BM, Zhao Y, Axon RN. US trends in prevalence, awareness, treatment, and control of hypertension, 1988–2008. J Am Med Assoc. 2010;303(20):2043–50.

47. Calhoun DA, Harding SM. Sleep and hypertension. Chest. 2010;138(2):434–43.

48. Young T, Peppard P, Palta M, et al. Population-based study of sleep-disordered breathing as a risk factor for hypertension. Arch Intern Med. 1997;157(15):1746–52.

49. Jean-Louis G, Zizi F, Clark LT, Brown CD, McFarlane SI. Obstructive sleep apnea and cardiovascular disease: role of the metabolic syndrome and its components. J Clin Sleep Med. 2008;4(3):261–72.

50. Dempsey JA, Veasey SC, Morgan BJ, O'Donnell CP. Pathophysiology of sleep apnea. Physiol Rev. 2010;90(1):47–112.

51. Lesske J, Fletcher EC, Bao G, Unger T. Hypertension caused by chronic intermittent hypoxia—influence of chemoreceptors and sympathetic nervous system. J Hypertens. 1997;15(12 Pt 2):1593–603.

52. Narkiewicz K, Somers VK. The sympathetic nervous system and obstructive sleep apnea: implications for hypertension. J Hypertens. 1997;15(12 Pt 2):1613–9.

53. Morgan BJ, Crabtree DC, Palta M, Skatrud JB. Combined hypoxia and hypercapnia evokes long-lasting sympathetic activation in humans. J Appl Physiol. 1995;79(1):205–13.

54. Guilleminault C, Motta J, Mihm F, Melvin K. Obstructive sleep apnea and cardiac index. Chest. 1986;89(3):331–4.

55. Schulz R, Mahmoudi S, Hattar K, et al. Enhanced release of superoxide from polymorphonuclear neutrophils in obstructive sleep apnea. Impact of continuous positive airway pressure therapy. Am J Respir Crit Care Med. 2000;162(2 Pt 1):566–70.

56. Kourembanas S, Marsden PA, McQuillan LP, Faller DV. Hypoxia induces endothelin gene expression and secretion in cultured human endothelium. J Clin Invest. 1991;88(3):1054–7.

57. Hartmann G, Tschop M, Fischer R, et al. High altitude increases circulating interleukin-6, interleukin-1 receptor antagonist and C-reactive protein. Cytokine. 2000;12(3):246–52.

58. Fletcher EC, Bao G, Li R. Renin activity and blood pressure in response to chronic episodic hypoxia. Hypertension. 1999;34(2):309–14.

59. Lavie P, Herer P, Hoffstein V. Obstructive sleep apnoea syndrome as a risk factor for hypertension: population study. Br Med J. 2000;320(7233):479–82.

60. Floras JS, Bradley TD. Treating obstructive sleep apnea: is there more to the story than 2 millimeters of mercury? Hypertension. 2007;50(2):289–91.

61. Buda AJ, Pinsky MR, Ingels Jr NB, Daughters GT, Stinson EB, Alderman EL. Effect of intrathoracic pressure on left ventricular performance. N Engl J Med. 1979;301(9):453–9.

62. Somers VK, Dyken ME, Skinner JL. Autonomic and hemodynamic responses and interactions during the Mueller maneuver in humans. J Auton Nerv Syst. 1993;44(2–3):253–9.

63. Otto ME, Belohlavek M, Romero-Corral A, et al. Comparison of cardiac structural and functional changes in obese otherwise healthy adults with versus without obstructive sleep apnea. Am J Cardiol. 2007;99(9):1298–302.

64. Romero-Corral A, Somers VK, Pellikka PA, et al. Decreased right and left ventricular myocardial performance in obstructive sleep apnea. Chest. 2007;132(6):1863–70.

65. Arias MA, Garcia-Rio F, Alonso-Fernandez A, Mediano O, Martinez I, Villamor J. Obstructive sleep apnea syndrome affects left ventricular diastolic function: effects of nasal continuous positive airway pressure in men. Circulation. 2005;112(3):375–83.

66. Sampol G, Romero O, Salas A, et al. Obstructive sleep apnea and thoracic aorta dissection. Am J Respir Crit Care Med. 2003;168(12):1528–31.

67. O'Brien E, Sheridan J, O'Malley K. Dippers and non-dippers. Lancet. 1988;2(8607):397.

68. Ohkubo T, Hozawa A, Yamaguchi J, et al. Prognostic significance of the nocturnal decline in blood pressure in individuals with and without high 24-h blood pressure: the Ohasama study. J Hypertens. 2002;20(11):2183–9.
69. Lavie L. Obstructive sleep apnoea syndrome-an oxidative stress disorder. Sleep Med Rev. 2003;7(1):35–51.
70. Ip MS, Lam B, Chan LY, et al. Circulating nitric oxide is suppressed in obstructive sleep apnea and is reversed by nasal continuous positive airway pressure. Am J Respir Crit Care Med. 2000;162(6):2166–71.
71. Nieto FJ, Young TB, Lind BK, et al. Association of sleep-disordered breathing, sleep apnea, and hypertension in a large community-based study. Sleep Heart Health Study. J Am Med Assoc. 2000;283(14):1829–36.
72. Peppard PE, Young T, Palta M, Skatrud J. Prospective study of the association between sleep-disordered breathing and hypertension. N Engl J Med. 2000;342(19):1378–84.
73. Somers VK, White DP, Amin R, et al. Sleep apnea and cardiovascular disease: an American Heart Association/American College of Cardiology Foundation Scientific Statement from the American Heart Association Council for High Blood Pressure Research Professional Education Committee, Council on Clinical Cardiology, Stroke Council, and Council on Cardiovascular Nursing. J Am Coll Cardiol. 2008;52(8):686–717.
74. Johns MW. A new method for measuring daytime sleepiness: the Epworth sleepiness scale. Sleep. 1991;14(6):540–5.
75. Netzer NC, Stoohs RA, Netzer CM, Clark K, Strohl KP. Using the Berlin questionnaire to identify patients at risk for the sleep apnea syndrome. Ann Intern Med. 1999;131(7):485–91.
76. Levendowski DJ, Olmstead EM, Popovich D, Carper D, Berka C, Westbrook PR. Assessment of obstructive sleep apnea risk and severity in truck drivers: validation of a screening questionnaire. Sleep Diagnosis Ther. 2007;2(2):20–6.
77. The American Academy of Sleep Medicine (Practice Parameters). http://www.aasmnet.org/practiceparameters.htm. Accessed August 24, 2011.
78. Noda A, Nakata S, Koike Y, et al. Continuous positive airway pressure improves daytime baroreflex sensitivity and nitric oxide production in patients with moderate to severe obstructive sleep apnea syndrome. Hypertens Res. 2007;30(8):669–76.
79. Bazzano LA, Khan Z, Reynolds K, He J. Effect of nocturnal nasal continuous positive airway pressure on blood pressure in obstructive sleep apnea. Hypertension. 2007;50(2):417–23.
80. Logan AG, Tkacova R, Perlikowski SM, et al. Refractory hypertension and sleep apnoea: effect of CPAP on blood pressure and baroreflex. Eur Respir J. 2003;21(2):241–7.
81. Barbe F, Duran-Cantolla J, Capote F, et al. Long-term effect of continuous positive airway pressure in hypertensive patients with sleep apnea. Am J Respir Crit Care Med. 2010;181(7):718–26.
82. Gotsopoulos H, Kelly JJ, Cistulli PA. Oral appliance therapy reduces blood pressure in obstructive sleep apnea: a randomized, controlled trial. Sleep. 2004;27(5):934–41.
83. Yu S, Liu F, Wang Q, et al. Effect of revised UPPP surgery on ambulatory BP in sleep apnea patients with hypertension and oropharyngeal obstruction. Clin Exp Hypertens. 2010;32(1):49–53.
84. Calhoun DA, Jones D, Textor S, et al. Resistant hypertension: diagnosis, evaluation, and treatment. A scientific statement from the American Heart Association Professional Education Committee of the Council for High Blood Pressure Research. Hypertension. 2008;51(6):1403–19.
85. Pratt-Ubunama MN, Nishizaka MK, Boedefeld RL, Cofield SS, Harding SM, Calhoun DA. Plasma aldosterone is related to severity of obstructive sleep apnea in subjects with resistant hypertension. Chest. 2007;131(2):453–9.
86. Calhoun DA, Nishizaka MK, Zaman MA, Harding SM. Aldosterone excretion among subjects with resistant hypertension and symptoms of sleep apnea. Chest. 2004;125(1):112–7.
87. Haffner SM, Lehto S, Ronnemaa T, Pyorala K, Laakso M. Mortality from coronary heart disease in subjects with type 2 diabetes and in nondiabetic subjects with and without prior myocardial infarction. N Engl J Med. 1998;339(4):229–34.

88. Selvin E, Marinopoulos S, Berkenblit G, et al. Meta-analysis: glycosylated hemoglobin and cardiovascular disease in diabetes mellitus. Ann Intern Med. 2004;141(6):421–31.

89. Pandey A, Demede M, Zizi F, et al. Sleep apnea and diabetes: insights into the emerging epidemic. Curr Diab Rep. 2011;11(1):35–40.

90. Demede M, Pandey A, Zizi F, et al. Resistant hypertension and obstructive sleep apnea in the primary-care setting. Int J Hypertens. 2011;2011:340929.

91. Jean-Louis G, Zizi F, Brown D, Ogedegbe G, Borer J, McFarlane S. Obstructive sleep apnea and cardiovascular disease: evidence and underlying mechanisms. Minerva Pneumol. 2009 Dec; 48(4):277–293.

Chapter 6
Resistant Hypertension: Etiology, Evaluation and Management

Oladipupo Olafiranye, Sidrah Mahmud, Ferdinand Zizi,
Samy I. McFarlane, Girardin Jean-louis, and Gbenga Ogedegbe

Definition and Prevalence

Resistant hypertension is defined as a failure to achieve goal blood pressure (BP) with maximum tolerated doses of three antihypertensive drugs including a diuretic or control of BP with 4 or more antihypertensive drugs of different classes at optimal doses [1–3]. The goal BP is 140/90 for most hypertensive patients and 130/80 for those with diabetes, renal insufficiency, or coronary heart disease [3]. The diagnosis of resistant hypertension requires use of good BP technique to confirm persistently elevated BP levels. Pseudoresistance due to patient nonadherence with medication, physician nonadherence with hypertension guidelines or underdosing, and white coat hypertension must be excluded. This condition often indicates the presence of secondary causes of hypertension. Although the true prevalence of resistance hypertension is currently unknown, population studies and clinical trials suggest that 20–35 % of hypertensive population have resistant hypertension [4–6].

O. Olafiranye
Division of Cardiology, Department of Medicine, SUNY-Downstate Medical Center, Brooklyn, NY, USA

S. Mahmud • F. Zizi • G. Jean-louis, Ph.D.
Department of Medicine, Sleep Disorder and Disparity Centers, SUNY Downstate Medical Center, 450 Clarkson Avenue, Box 1199, Brooklyn, NY 11203-2098, USA
e-mail: girardin.jean-louis@downstate.edu

S.I. McFarlane, M.D., M.P.H., M.B.A.
Division of Endocrinology, Diabetes and Hypertension, Department of Medicine, SUNY-Downstate and Kings County Hospital, Brooklyn, NY, USA
e-mail: Samy.McFarlane@downstate.edu

G. Ogedegbe, M.D.(⊠)
Division of General Internal Medicine, Department of Medicine, Center for Healthful Behavior Change, New York University School of Medicine, New York, NY, USA
e-mail: Olugbenga.Ogedegbe@nyumc.org

S.I. McFarlane and G.L. Bakris (eds.), *Diabetes and Hypertension: Evaluation and Management*, Contemporary Diabetes, DOI 10.1007/978-1-60327-357-2_6,
© Springer Science+Business Media New York 2012

According to the 2002 World Health Report, uncontrolled BP is the most common attributable risk for death worldwide, being responsible for about 50 % of coronary heart disease and 62 % of stroke [7, 8].

Etiology of Resistant Hypertension

A number of factors and/or mechanisms are involved in the maintenance of normal BP. When these mechanisms become dysfunctional, individuals with hypertension may experience resistance to treatment. Factors that are believed to play a role in the development of resistant hypertension include patient characteristics, alcohol and dietary salt, medications, and secondary causes of hypertension (Table 6.1). Of note, in most cases multiple factors are thought to be responsible for uncontrolled BP.

Table 6.1 Factors contributing to true resistant hypertension

1. Patient characteristics
    - Age
    - Obesity
    - Female gender
    - Black race
    - Genetics
2. Dietary salt
3. Alcohol
4. Medications
    - Nonsteroidal anti-inflammatory drugs
    - Selective COX-2 inhibitors
    - Illicit drugs (cocaine, amphetamines, etc.)
    - Stimulants (amphetamine, methylphenidate, etc.)
    - Sympathomimetics (decongestants, diet pills)
    - Oral contraceptive
    - Erythropoietin
    - Cyclosporin
    - Natural Licorice
5. Secondary causes of hypertension
    - Obstructive sleep apnea
    - Renal parenchymal disease
    - Renal artery stenosis
    - Primary aldosteronism
    - Pheochromocytoma
    - Cushing's disease
    - Hyperparathyroidism
    - Aortic coarctation
    - Intracranial tumor

Factors Contributing to True Resistance to Treatment

Patient Characteristics

Certain patient characteristics have been shown to be associated with resistant hypertension. These include older age (>65 years), obesity, female sex, black race, and individual genetic makeup. Increasing age is associated with arterial stiffening, which results in difficult to control systolic BP [9, 10]. Obesity, which is also common among patients with resistant hypertension [11], has been associated with need for an increased number of antihypertensive medications, more severe hypertension, and an increased likelihood that achieving goal BP cannot be achieved [9, 12]. The mechanisms by which obesity contributes to difficult-to-treat hypertension are complex and not completely understood. Increased sympathetic activity, impaired sodium excretion, activation of the renin–angiotensin–aldosterone system, increased aldosterone sensitivity related to visceral adiposity, and obstructive sleep apnea have all been implicated as potential mechanisms [13–16].

Genetic factors may also contribute to the development of resistant hypertension. Studies have shown that generally African Americans, who have shown genetically "low renin" levels, have enhanced responses to calcium channel blockers and thiazide and lower responses to direct renin inhibitors, angiotensin-converting enzyme (ACE) inhibitors, and angiotensin receptor blockers (ARBs). Genetic differences in acetylation kinetics of hydralazine can affect the dose required to lower BP. Therefore, identification of genes that influence resistance to current antihypertensive agents might be of therapeutic target in the nearest future.

Dietary Salt and Alcohol

Excess dietary salt intake is a major factor that plays an important role in the development of resistant hypertension in most cases. It can directly increase BP by causing volume overload/expansion [17] or can indirectly increase BP by blunting the blood pressure-lowering effect of most classes of antihypertensive agents [18–20]. These effects are most pronounced in salt-sensitive patients; these include renal disease patients, individuals of African American background, and the elderly [21].

Modest alcohol intake does not usually increase BP. However, heavy alcohol intake is associated with both an increased risk of developing hypertension as well as resistance to hypertensive therapy [3]. It has been suggested that large amount of alcohol (3 or more drinks/day) have a dose-related effect on BP, in both hypertensive and normotensive individuals [3].

Medications

A number of pharmacological agents can produce transient or sustained increase in BP and contribute to treatment resistance [22] (Table 6.1). However, the effects of these agents on BP vary from one individual to another, with most people manifesting little or no effect, and few experiencing severe BP elevations. Nonsteroidal anti-inflammatory agents (NSAIDs) such as aspirin and Ibuprofen are probably the most common medication-related cause of uncontrolled BP [22, 23]. NSAIDs are associated with modest but predictable increases in BP [23] and can blunt the blood pressure lowering effect of several antihypertensive agents, including ACE inhibitors, ARBs, β-blockers, and diuretics [24, 25]. Selective cyclooxygenase-2 (COX-2) inhibitors have also been reported to have similar effects [26, 27]. These effects presumably occur subsequent to inhibition of renal prostaglandin production, especially prostaglandin E2 and prostaglandin I2, leading to sodium and fluid retention. It has been shown that elderly patients, diabetics, and patients with CKD are at increased risk of manifesting these adverse effects. Several other medications have also been implicated in the etiology of resistant hypertension as listed in Table 6.1.

Secondary Causes of Hypertension

Secondary causes of hypertension are relatively common among patients with resistant hypertension and should always be considered. Studies suggest that about 5–10 % of resistant hypertension patients have identifiable cause, although the true prevalence of secondary causes remains unknown [28, 29]. The common secondary causes include renal parenchymal disease, obstructive sleep apnea, primary aldosteronism, and renal artery stenosis. Less common causes include pheochromocytoma, hyperparathyroidism, hypoparathyroidism, Cushing's syndrome, aortic coarctation, and intracranial tumors (Table 6.1). Description of the signs and symptoms, diagnostic procedures, and treatment of these secondary causes of hypertension is beyond the scope of this chapter.

Factors Contributing to Pseudoresistance

Pseudoresistant hypertension refers to uncontrolled BP or elevated BP readings as a result of some preventable factors, other than those described above. Such factors include:

1. Poor BP measuring technique
2. Poor patient adherence to prescribed medications
3. Poor physician adherence to hypertension guidelines
4. Physician inertia—failure to increase dose or add medication when not at goal
5. White coat effect—clinic BP readings are consistently higher than out-of-office readings. This is usually related to anxiety when in doctors' office

Evaluation of Patients with Resistant Hypertension

Accurate diagnosis of resistant hypertension and identification of related causes can be made through detailed medical history, thorough physical examination, appropriate BP measurement technique, and laboratory testing. It is important to note that the etiology of treatment resistance is multifactorial.

Medical History

A detailed medical history should be obtained from patients with suspected resistant hypertension. Specific questions regarding current medications use, duration of use, and treatment adherence should be asked. Information about herbal and over-the-counter medications, medication adverse effects, and symptoms of possible secondary causes of hypertension should be sought. Patients should also be asked about their adherence to prescribed medications. Information regarding adherence can also be obtained from family members with the permission of the patient.

Blood Pressure Measurement

Proper BP measurement technique is essential for accurate diagnosis of resistant hypertension. BP should be taken using appropriate cuff size and with the patient sitting quietly in a chair and his or her back supported for 5 min before taking the measurement. The correct cuff size should encircle at least 80 % of the arm, and during measurement it should be at the level of the heart [30]. The BP should be measured carefully in both arms, and the arm with the higher pressures generally should be used to make future measurements. The average of a minimum of two readings taken at 1 min intervals is generally advised to be taken as patients BP.

Physical Examination

A thorough physical examination including weight and height are necessary in the identification of causes of true resistant hypertension and secondary causes of hypertension. Physical signs of end organ damage may also be discovered during physical examination. Fundoscopic examination is recommended to document the presence and severity of retinopathy.

Ambulatory Blood Pressure Monitoring

Among patients with suspected white-coat hypertension, reliable assessment of out-of-office BP values is required. This is best accomplished with the use of 24-h ambulatory BP monitoring. Alternatively, out-of-office patient self-assessments with use of manual or automated BP monitors can be relied on. If a significant white-coat effect is confirmed, out-of-office measurements should be relied on to adjust treatment [31].

Other Tests

Various tests can be performed to identify secondary causes of hypertension. However description of these diagnostic procedures is beyond the scope of this chapter.

Treatment

Management of resistant hypertension can be broadly divided into nonpharmacological and pharmacological interventions. Since the etiology of this condition is almost always multifactorial, a multidisciplinary treatment approach including doctors, pharmacists, nurse case manager, and nutritionist can improve treatment outcome. Both nonpharmacological and pharmacological treatment modalities tailored toward the identified etiologies are often required to achieve the goal BP.

Nonpharmacological Interventions

Appropriate lifestyle changes such as regular exercise, weight loss, moderate alcohol intake, low-salt diet, and medication adherence should be reinforced. The current guidelines suggest that dietary sodium for a hypertensive person should be <100 mmol per day (2.4 g sodium or 6 g sodium chloride) [3]. These are applicable to all patients with resistant hypertension, although salt-sensitive patients may require even lower amounts of sodium. Alcohol intake in all hypertensive patients should be limited to no more than 1 oz (2 drinks) of ethanol a day for most men and 0.5 oz (1 drink) of ethanol a day for women.

Pharmacological Interventions

Modification of the antihypertensive regimen is often required for most patients with resistant hypertension despite adequate nonpharmacological interventions.

It is important to withdraw other medications that may interfere with BP control, particularly NSAIDs, before adjusting antihypertensive regimen. In situations where this is clinically difficult, the lowest effective dose of such medications should be used with subsequent down titration whenever possible. It is well known that suboptimal dosing regimen and inappropriate antihypertensive drug combinations are the most common causes of uncontrolled hypertension [3]. Hence, medication dosages should be optimized and antihypertensive agents of different mechanisms of action should be combined. The recommendation of combination therapy is based on additive antihypertensive benefit. However, this recommendation is largely empiric, since there is little data assessing the efficacy of specific combinations of three or more drugs. Patient characteristics (age, race, comorbidities) usually determine the best combination of agents needed to achieve goal BP. However, a combination of thiazide diuretic, ACE inhibitor, and ARBs are effective for most patients.

If the goal BP is not achieved with full doses of four appropriately combined drugs, other agents such as centrally acting alpha-agonists (clonidine and methyldopa) and potent vasodilators (hydralazine or minoxidil) are needed to control the BP; however, adverse effects of these medications limit their use. If a β (beta)-antagonist is required for the added benefit of heart rate control, the combined α (alpha)–β (beta)-antagonists are preferred because of their greater antihypertensive effects [32]. Diuretic is mandatory for all patients with resistant hypertension in cases where there is no contraindication. Research has shown that BP control is improved by adding a diuretic, increasing the dose of the diuretic, or changing the class of prescribed diuretic based on the underlying renal function [33]. This is especially true for most patients and elderly patients in particular, since inappropriate volume expansion contributes to treatment resistance [34]. Although long-acting thiazide diuretic is commonly used for BP control, chlorthalidone has been shown to have superior efficacy and is therefore the preferred diuretic agent for resistant hypertension. Recently, another class of agents, endothelial receptor antagonists (ERA) proved effective in the treatment of resistant hypertension. However, there are limited evidence in support of their use, and therefore not recommended at this time.

Finally, for those patients with uncontrolled BP with four or more medications lasting longer than 6 months, referral to a hypertension specialist is advisable [1]. Also, if a specific secondary cause of hypertension is identified or suspected, referral to the appropriate specialist for further evaluation and management is recommended.

References

1. Calhoun DA, Jones D, Textor S, Goff DC, Murphy TP, Toto RD, et al. Resistant hypertension: diagnosis, evaluation, and treatment: a scientific statement from the American Heart Association Professional Education Committee of the Council for High Blood Pressure Research. Circulation. 2008;117(25):e510–26.
2. Calhoun DA, Jones D, Textor S, Goff DC, Murphy TP, Toto RD, et al. Resistant hypertension: diagnosis, evaluation, and treatment: a scientific statement from the American Heart Association Professional Education Committee of the Council for High Blood Pressure Research. Hypertension. 2008;51(6):1403–19.

3. Chobanian AV, Bakris GL, Black HR, et al. Seventh report of the joint national committee on prevention, detection, evaluation, and treatment of high blood pressure. Hypertension. 2003;42:1206–52.
4. ALLHAT Officers and Coordinators for the ALLHAT Collaborative Research Group. The Antihypertensive and Lipid-Lowering Treatment to Prevent Heart Attack Trial. Major outcomes in high-risk hypertensive patients randomized to angiotensin-converting enzyme inhibitor or calcium channel blocker vs diuretic: the Antihypertensive and Lipid-Lowering Treatment to Prevent Heart Attack Trial (ALLHAT). J Am Med Assoc. 2002;288:2981–97.
5. Dahlof B, Devereux RB, Kjeldsen SE, et al. Cardiovascular morbidity and mortality in the losartan intervention for endpoint reduction in hypertension study (LIFE): a randomised trial against atenolol. Lancet. 2002;359:995–1003.
6. Pepine CJ, Handberg EM, Cooper-DeHoff RM, et al. A calcium antagonist vs a non-calcium antagonist hypertension treatment strategy for patients with coronary artery disease: The International Verapamil-Trandolapril Study (INVEST): a randomized controlled trial. J Am Med Assoc. 2003;290:2805–16.
7. World Health Organization. World health report 2002: reducing risks, promoting healthy life. Geneva, Switzerland: World Health Organization; 2002.
8. Sarafidis PA, Bakris GL. Resistant hypertension: an overview of evaluation and treatment. J Am Coll Cardiol. 2008;52(22):1749–57.
9. Lloyd-Jones DM, Evans JC, Larson MG, O'Donnell CJ, Rocella EJ, Levy D. Differential control of systolic and diastolic blood pressure: factors associated with lack of blood pressure control in the community. Hypertension. 2000;36:594–9.
10. Cushman WC, Ford CE, Cutler JA, Margolis KL, Davis BR, Grimm RH, et al. Success and predictors of blood pressure control in diverse North American settings: the Antihypertensive and Lipid-Lowering and Treatment to Prevent Heart Attack Trial (ALLHAT). J Clin Hypertens. 2002;4:393–404.
11. Nishizaka MK, Pratt-Ubunama M, Zaman MA, Cofield S, Calhoun DA. Validity of plasma aldosterone-to-renin activity ratio in African American and white subjects with resistant hypertension. Am J Hypertens. 2005;18:805–12.
12. Bramlage P, Pittrow D, Wittchen H-U, Kirch W, Boehler S, Lehnert H, et al. Hypertension in overweight and obese primary care patients is highly prevalent and poorly controlled. Am J Hypertens. 2004;17:904–10.
13. Hall JE. The kidney, hypertension, and obesity. Hypertension. 2003;41(Part 2):625–33.
14. Morris MJ. Cardiovascular and metabolic effects of obesity. Clin Exp Pharmacol Physiol. 2008;35:416–9.
15. Sarafidis PA. Obesity, insulin resistance and kidney disease risk: insights into the relationship. Curr Opin Nephrol Hypertens. 2008;17:450–6.
16. Wong C, Marwick TH. Obesity cardiomyopathy: pathogenesis and pathophysiology. Nat Clin Pract Cardiovasc Med. 2007;4:436–43.
17. Sarafidis PA, Bakris GL. State of hypertension management in the United States: confluence of risk factors and the prevalence of resistant hypertension. J Clin Hypertens (Greenwich). 2008;10:130–9.
18. He FJ, MacGregor GA. Effect of longer-term modest salt reduction on blood pressure. Cochrane Database Syst Rev. 2004;3:CD004937.
19. Luft FC, Weinberger MH. Review of salt restriction and the response to antihypertensive drugs: satellite symposium on calcium antagonists. Hypertension. 1988;11(Suppl I):I-229–32.
20. Weinberger MH, Cohen SJ, Miller JZ, Luft FC, Grim CE, Fineberg NS. Dietary sodium restriction as adjunctive treatment of hypertension. J Am Med Assoc. 1988;259:2561–5.
21. Boudville N, Ward S, Benaroia M, House AA. Increased sodium intake correlates with greater use of antihypertensive agents by subjects with chronic kidney disease. Am J Hypertens. 2005;18:1300–5.
22. Grossman E, Messerli FH. Secondary hypertension: interfering substances. J Clin Hypertens (Greenwich). 2008;10:556–66.

23. Johnson AG, Nguyen TV, Day RO. Do nonsteroidal anti-inflammatory drugs affect blood pressure? a meta-analysis. Ann Intern Med. 1994;121:289–300.
24. Radack KL, Deck CC, Bloomfield SS. Ibuprofen interferes with the efficacy of antihypertensive drugs. A randomized, double-blind, placebo-controlled trial of ibuprofen compared with acetaminophen. Ann Intern Med. 1987;107:628–35.
25. Conlin PR, Moore TJ, Swartz SL, Barr E, Gazdick L, Fletcher C, et al. Effect of indomethacin on blood pressure lowering by captopril and losartan in hypertensive patients. Hypertension. 2000;36:461–5.
26. Whelton A, White WB, Bello AE, Puma JA, Fort JG. SUCCESS-VII investigators. Effects of celecoxib and rofecoxib on blood pressure and edema in patients > or =65 years of age with systemic hypertension and osteoarthritis. Am J Cardiol. 2002;90:959–63.
27. White WB, Kent J, Taylor A, Verburg KM, Lefkowith JB, Whelton A. Effects of celecoxib on ambulatory blood pressure in hypertensive patients on ACE inhibitors. Hypertension. 2002;39:929–34.
28. Yakovlevitch M, Black HR. Resistant hypertension in a tertiary care clinic. Arch Intern Med. 1991;151:1786–92.
29. Garg JP, Elliott WJ, Folker A, Izhar M, Black HR. Resistant hypertension revisited: a comparison of two university-based cohorts. Am J Hypertens. 2005;18:619–26.
30. Pickering TG, Hall JE, Appel LJ, Falkner BE, Graves J, Hill MN, et al. Recommendations of blood pressure measurement in humans and experimental animals. Part 1: blood pressure measurement in humans. A statement for Professionals from the Subcommittee of Professional and Public Education of the American Heart Association Council on High Blood Pressure Research. Circulation. 2005;111:697–716.
31. Niiranen TJ, Kantola IM, Vesalainen R, Johansson J, Ruuska MJ. A comparison of home measurement and ambulatory monitoring of blood pressure in the adjustment of antihypertensive treatment. Am J Hypertens. 2006;19:468–74.
32. Townsend RR, DiPette DJ, Goodman R, Blumfield D, Cronin R, Gradman A, et al. Combined alpha/beta-blockade versus beta 1-selective blockade in essential hypertension in black and white patients. Clin Pharmacol Ther. 1990;48:665–75.
33. Taler SJ, Textor SC, Augustine JE. Resistant hypertension: comparing hemodynamic management to specialist care. Hypertension. 2002;39:982–8.
34. Vlase HL, Panagopoulos G, Michelis MF. Effectiveness of furosemide in uncontrolled hypertension in the elderly: role of renin profiling. Am J Hypertens. 2003;16:187–93.

Chapter 7
Diabetes and Cardiovascular Disease

Mariana Garcia-Touza and James R. Sowers

Pathogenesis of Atherosclerosis in Diabetes

Cardiovascular disease (CVD) is the leading cause of premature mortality in diabetes. The role of diabetes as a contributing factor to CVD becomes clear after the publication of the 20 years of surveillance of the Framingham cohort study in 1979. In this cohort, a twofold to threefold increased risk of clinical atherosclerotic disease was reported in patients with prior evidence of diabetes [1]. CVDs, morbidity, and mortality for diabetic women were higher than that for nondiabetic men.

The pathogenesis of CVD in diabetes is multifactorial and can be affected by metabolic factors such as insulin resistance, increased release of cytokines and bioactive mediators by the adipose tissue, chronic inflammation, and oxidative stress leading to endothelial dysfunction and inappropriate activation of the renin–angiotensin–aldosterone system (RAAS). There is emerging evidence that increasing obesity in young adults contributes to parallel increases in CVD and chronic renal disease in persons with cardiorenal syndrome (CRS) as well those with type 2 diabetes [2]. Thus, in states of obesity and insulin resistance there is a constellation of interactive cardiac and renal risk factors, including hypertension, metabolic dyslipidemia, microalbuminuria and/or reduced renal function, increased systemic

M. Garcia-Touza
Division of Endocrinology, Diabetes and Metabolism, Department of Internal Medicine, University of Missouri-Columbia School of Medicine, Columbia, MO, USA

J.R. Sowers, M.D. (✉)
Division of Endocrinology, Diabetes and Metabolism, Department of Internal Medicine, University of Missouri-Columbia School of Medicine, Columbia, MO, USA

Harry S. Truman Memorial Veterans' Hospital, Columbia, MO, USA
e-mail: sowersj@health.missouri.edu

S.I. McFarlane and G.L. Bakris (eds.), *Diabetes and Hypertension: Evaluation and Management*, Contemporary Diabetes, DOI 10.1007/978-1-60327-357-2_7, © Springer Science+Business Media New York 2012

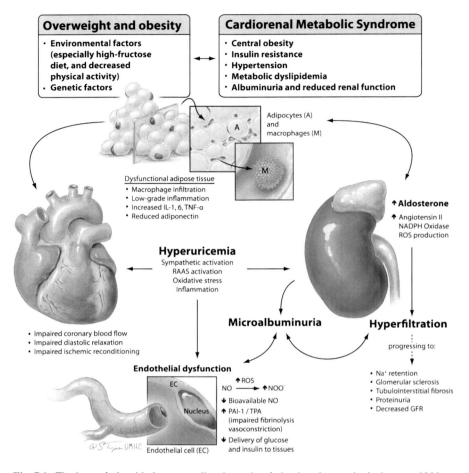

Fig. 7.1 The interrelationship between adiposity and maladaptive changes in the heart and kidney in the cardiorenal system. *GFR* glomerular filtration rate, *IL* interleukin, *PAI* plasminogen activator inhibitor, *RASS* renin–angiotensin–aldosterone system, *ROS* reactive oxygen species, *TNF* tumor necrosis factor, *PTA* tissue plasminogen activator

inflammation, oxidative stress, and hypercoagulability that enhance CVD risk (Fig. 7.1). With the development of pancreatic dysfunction and hyperglycemia, these patients are of even greater risk for CVD [1–4].

Metabolic Factors. Metabolic imbalances related to CRS and diabetes mellitus include hyperglycemia and its derivatives, advanced glycation end products (AGEs), increased levels of free fatty acids (FFAs), reduced levels of adiponectin, and lipoprotein abnormalities. Hyperglycemia increases oxidative stress diminishing the levels of nitric oxide (NO), which leads to endothelial cell apoptosis, impaired endothelial mediated vascular relaxation, and increased vascular glycation abnormalities [3, 4]. In addition, hyperglycemia increases glycation of lipoproteins and alters lipid metabolism leading to activation of protein kinase C and tumor necrosis factor alpha (TNF-alpha). It can also alter insulin signaling, increase endothelial cell adhesion molecule gene expression, and stimulate inflammation and smooth muscle migration and proliferation [5, 6]. High levels of FFAs are also detrimental, leading to increased oxidative stress and diminished endothelial cell NO synthesis. These glycation abnormalities can also impair fibrinolysis by increasing concentrations of plasminogen activator inhibitor (PAI-1) [7, 8].

FFAs are believed to play a major role in increased hepatic gluconeogenesis and overproduction of triglyceride-rich very low-density lipoprotein, which in turn lead to higher levels of atherogenic low-density lipoproteins (LDLs) and decreased high-density lipoproteins (HDLs). The abnormal lipoprotein metabolism negatively influences endothelial function and promotes the atherogenic process.

Lipoprotein abnormalities are usually seen in people with CRS and diabetes and include an elevation of triglycerides and increased small dense low HDL. There is no difference in the LDL levels, but the particles are smaller, more dense, and more atherogenic [9].

Visceral Adiposity. Adipocytes are an active endocrine and paracrine organ and are recognized as a rich source of pro-inflammatory mediators that contribute to vascular injury, insulin resistance, and atherogenesis [2]. These adipokines include TNF-alpha, interleukin 6 (IL-6), leptin, plasminogen activator inhibitor-1, resistin, and C-reactive protein [10]. Circulating adipokine levels are elevated in an insulin-resistant state and visceral/intra-abdominal fat produces inflammatory adipokines in greater amounts than other fat depots. On the other hand, adiponectin, which is also produced by adipocytes, increases fat oxidation, improves endothelial-mediated vasorelaxation and insulin sensitivity [11]. This hormone is negatively regulated by glucocorticoids and TNF-alpha and positively by insulin metabolic signaling [12]. Adiponectin levels are decreased in obesity and are inversely correlated to insulin-resistant states and high-sensitivity C-reactive protein (CRP) levels. Patients with the CRS, diabetes, and coronary heart disease have lower adiponectin levels [13].

Oxidation/Glycoxidation. Diabetes can affect the generation of oxygen-centered free radicals by glucose-dependent and -independent mechanisms. Auto-oxidation of glucose can generate oxygen-centered free radicals. Cellular oxidation of glucose generates excess reactive oxygen species in mitochondria. These free radicals can lead to increased lipid peroxidation in lipoproteins. The arterial wall can be modified by the process of glycation driven by hyperglycemia and associated increases in oxidative stress, a process called glycoxidation [14, 15]. This process generates AGEs that attack proteins and lipids which lead to vascular inflammation, remodeling, and hypertrophy.

Inflammation. This is a key player in the initiation and progression of atherosclerosis [16]. AGE-mediated cytokine release is associated with overproduction of inflammatory growth factors such as platelet-dependent growth factor, insulin-like growth factor-1, granulocyte/monocyte colony-stimulating factor, and transforming growth factor alpha and beta. An additional inflammatory phenomenon involves increased formation of immune complexes and subsequent activation of macrophages by these complexes leading to release of CRP. The increase in immune complexes can also contribute to plaque rupture and acute coronary events [17, 18].

Endothelial dysfunction. Diabetes and insulin-resistant states such as CRS often manifest altered expression of adhesion molecules that affect thrombosis and increased vascular permeability. There is also an impaired response to endothelium NO-dependent vasodilators [2]. Insulin has a dose- and time-dependent effect of increasing vasodilatation in animal models and humans [2, 19]. The action of insulin appeared to be mediated by the ability to produce NO and to diminish its destruction. AGEs and oxidation products have the ability to destroy endothelial cell derived NO. This mechanism is an important contributor to the vasodilatation impairment seen in the CRS and diabetes. Evidence suggests that inflammatory adipokines may negatively influence endothelial function through their pro-inflammatory properties. On the other hand, adiponectin, which is reduced in the CRS and diabetes, normally promotes NO-mediated vasorelaxation.

Diabetes and the CRS are associated with a pro-thrombotic state reflecting changes in both thrombosis and fibrinolysis. There is an increase in factor VII activity related, among other things, to elevated postprandial hyperlipidemia. PAI-1 overexpression may be attributable to direct effects of insulin and increased inflammation. Increases in platelet aggregation have all been described in diabetes [15]. All of these abnormalities contribute to systemic oxidation, inflammation, hypercoagulability, and enhanced platelet adhesion and aggregation [2, 15].

Activation of the RAAS. The CRS and diabetes are often associated with inappropriate activation of the RAAS [20]. Elevations in angiotensin II and aldosterone have been shown to promote an impairment in systemic insulin metabolic signaling that leads to endothelial dysfunction and myocardial functional abnormalities [21]. Enhanced activation of the RAAS and increases in oxidative stress can cause decreased mitochondrial biogenesis and increased apoptosis and accumulation of lipids in the heart. Recent evidence suggests that impaired myocardial mitochondrial biogenesis, fatty acid metabolism, and antioxidant defense mechanisms lead to diminished cardiac substrate flexibility and diastolic dysfunction [22]. The maladaptive interaction of factors such as hypertension, insulin resistance, dyslipidemia, microalbuminuria, and reduced renal function has been called the CRS [23]. Figure 7.1 shows the interrelationship between adiposity and maladaptive changes in the heart and kidney in patients with insulin resistance. Atherosclerosis and myocardial dysfunction are increased in persons with insulin resistance and diabetes type 1 and 2. However, the exact mechanism and potential benefits of correcting these abnormalities are still under investigation.

Evidence-Based Glycemic Medical Treatment

The publications of the Diabetes Control and Complications Trial (DCCT) in 1993 and United Kingdom Prospective Diabetes Study (UKPDS) in 1998 helped shape the management of diabetes in recent years [24, 25]. Both studies showed a significant reduction in microvascular disease with intensive glucose control and reduction of hemoglobin A1C of 7%. Unfortunately, these studies were not able to demonstrate a benefit in reduction of myocardial infarction or macrovascular disease. The UKPDS involved intensive treatment of hyperglycemia in patients with newly diagnosed type 2 diabetes over a 10-year period. There is an absolute reduction in the risk of myocardial infarction of borderline significance (3%) with no significant reductions in any other macrovascular outcomes. There was also preliminary evidence that metformin treatment may reduce CVD events in the UKPDS.

The first study that showed a treatment benefit in the reduction of CVD in diabetes was the Steno-2 study published in 2003 [26]. This study was an intensified intervention aimed at multiple risk factors in patients with type 2 diabetes. This was a randomized study with implementation of behavior modification and pharmacologic therapy targeting hyperglycemia, hypertension, dyslipidemia, and microalbuminuria. The mean follow-up was 7.9 years and the study showed a reduction in the risk of cardiovascular and microvascular events by about 50%.

The lack of reduction of macrovascular disease evidence in the UKPDS study gave birth to the notion that a more aggressive approach targeting hemoglobin A1C below 7% would reduce CVD. This hypothesis was tested in three studies: the Veterans Administration Diabetes Trial (VADT), Action in Diabetes and Vascular Disease: Preterax and Diamicron Modified Release Controlled Evaluation (ADVANCE) and Action to Control Cardiovascular Risk in Diabetes (ACCORD). These studies were published in rapid succession over the second half of 2008 and the beginning of 2009. A total number of almost 25,000 type 2 diabetic patients were recruited in these trials to assess the effect of intensive glycemic control vs. conventional therapy on CVD endpoints [27].

The VADT was published in 2009. This study enrolled 1,791 military veterans with suboptimal response to therapy for type 2 diabetes. CVD risk factors were treated uniformly, and the patients were randomized into intensive therapy and standard therapy with an absolute reduction of hemoglobin A1C of 1.5 percentage points between the two groups. The primary outcome was a composite of myocardial infarction, stroke and death from CVD, and congestive heart failure, surgery for vascular disease, inoperable coronary disease, and amputation for ischemic gangrene. The median follow-up was 5.6 years with a reduction in the hemoglobin A1C in the intensive arm of 6.9%. The intensive glucose control in this study had no significant effect on the rates of major cardiovascular events or death. The study showed a reduction in the progression of albuminuria [28].

The ADVANCE trial was a study designed to answer the question whether intensifying glucose control to achieve an A1C of <6.5% would provide an additional benefit of reducing the risk of both micro- and macrovascular disease. The ADVANCE had also a blood pressure (BP) lowering arm in patients with type 2 diabetes. The aim of the BP arm was to establish whether routine provision of BP lowering therapy produced additional benefits in terms of macro- and microvascular disease, irrespective of the baseline BP. The trial enrolled over 10,000 patients from 20 countries in Asia, Europe, Australia, and North America with a median follow-up of 5 years. The hemoglobin A1C fell progressively in the intensive arm, reaching 6.5% in a period of 2–3 years duration. The study demonstrated that it is possible to safely achieve tight levels of glycemic control using conventional agents.

Unfortunately, there were no significant differences in the number of macrovascular events between the two groups during the trial. Again, there was a 14% relative risk reduction in microvascular events especially diabetic nephropathy. The BP arm of the ADVANCE trial ran for 4.3 years and showed that a combination of indapamide and perindopril reduced mortality, coronary events, and diabetic nephropathy regardless of the initial BP [29].

The ACCORD trial is the last of the three mega trials in glucose control and macrovascular disease. The study was published in 2008 and the hypothesis was to investigate whether intensive therapy targeting a hemoglobin A1C of 6% would reduce CVD events in patients with type 2 diabetes. This study randomized 10,251 patients and the hemoglobin A1C was reduced by 1.4% in the intensive therapy in a period of 4 months. Findings of higher mortality in the intensive therapy arm led to discontinuation of the study after a mean of 3.5 years of follow-up [30]. This study had identified a previously unrecognized harm of intensive glucose lowering in high-risk patient with type 2 diabetes. The intensive therapy group had higher rates of hypoglycemia, weight gain, and fluid retention. Patients in the two groups had similar exposure to cardiovascular protective interventions; BP levels were lower in the intensive therapy arm. The study suggested that patients in the intensive arm who had not had CVD and a hemoglobin A1C less than 8% may have had fewer fatal or nonfatal CVD events. Preliminary analysis of episodes of severe hypoglycemia and differences in the use of drugs, weight change, and other factors did not identify an explanation for the increase in mortality. Some hypothesized that the harm may be related to the speed and magnitude of reduction in the hemoglobin A1C level in the intensive group.

These three trials have demonstrated that, at least in the short term (3–5 years), aggressive glycemic control of hemoglobin A1C to 6–6.5% has no significant effect in reducing macrovascular disease. On the other hand, these trials showed a decline in CVD mortality in the diabetic population regardless of the glycemic control [31]. This reduction in CVD is related to the efforts made targeting other aspects of type 2 diabetes such as BP and cholesterol reduction with the knowledge that this will have a larger effect preventing macrovascular complications as evidenced in the STENO-2 trial and the Avoiding Cardiovascular Events in Combination Therapy in Patients Living with Systolic Hypertension (ACCOMPLISH) trial.

The Legacy Effects of Glycemic Control

The DCCT showed that intensive therapy aimed to achieve near normoglycemia reduces the risk of microvascular complications in type 1 diabetes. In this study, patients with new onset type 1 diabetes were randomly assigned to intensive vs. conventional therapy from 1983 to 1993. Ninety-three percent of these patients were followed until 2005 by the Epidemiology of Diabetes Interventions and Complications (EDIC) Study group. With a mean of 17 years of follow-up, the study showed that intense diabetes therapy reduced the risk of any CVD event by 42% and the risk of nonfatal myocardial infarction, stroke, or death from CVD by

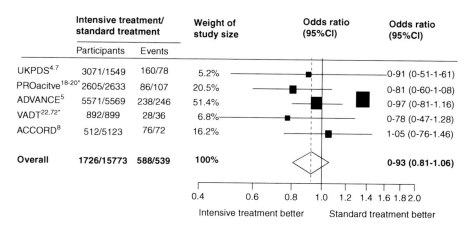

Fig. 7.2 Meta-analysis showed that intensive glycemic control resulted in 17% reduction in events of nonfatal myocardial infarction and 15% reduction in events of coronary heart disease

57%. Microalbuminuria and albuminuria were associated with a significant increase in the risk of CVD [32].

In the UKPDS study, patients with new onset type 2 diabetes who received intensive glucose therapy had a lower risk of microvascular complications. Post-trial monitoring of these patients was done through annual questionnaires. These patients were followed up for a period of 17 years. The differences in hemoglobin A1C level between groups were lost after the first year. Despite this early loss of glycemic differences, a continued reduction in microvascular risk and emergent reductions for myocardial infarction and death from any cause were observed in the post-trial follow-up [33]. This beneficial effect in the intensive arm, despite the loss of separation in the glycemic control, has been called the legacy effect (Fig. 7.2).

The concept of a glycemic legacy effect has been proposed based on the long-term follow-up of these studies. In both studies, the risk reduction for microvascular disease after almost 20 years of follow-up was fully retained despite the loss in the separation in hemoglobin A1C level between the two groups. Even more remarkable was the risk reduction for CVD (−57%, 95% CI 12–7%) in the DCCT and reduced risk of myocardial infarction of 15% in the UKPDS. This showed that the effect of tight glycemic control in newly diagnosed patients is equally beneficial in type 1 and type 2 diabetes.

On the other hand, the decrease in the incidence of nephropathy that was demonstrated in the ADVANCE and VADT trials might have long-term benefits on CVD. Patients with diabetic nephropathy have a 20% higher risk of macrovascular disease [34].

The gestalt emerging from these trials has a more favorable outcome on CVD with contemporary therapy in diabetic patients in recent years. This is related to a multiple targeted approach (BP, lipid, microalbuminuria, and antiplatelet therapy) and long-term follow-up effects of more rigorous glucose control. Indeed, a meta-analysis in 2009 of these prospective randomized controlled trials (Fig. 7.2) showed that intensive glycemic control resulted in 17% reduction in events of nonfatal myocardial infarction and a 15% reduction in events of coronary heart disease. Intensive glycemic control had no effect on events of stroke or all-cause mortality [35].

Conclusions and Recommendations

Intensive glycemic control early and late in diabetes significantly reduces the risk of microvascular complications. It may reduce the risk of CVD events as per long-term follow-up studies (EDIC/UKPDS follow-up). However, this approach will increase the risk of severe hypoglycemia and weight gain which may limit the magnitude of these benefits. It is now generally acknowledged that target hemoglobin A1C goal should be individualized based on duration of diabetes, age/life expectancy, comorbid conditions, known CVD or advanced microvascular complications, hypoglycemia unawareness, and individual patient considerations. More or less stringent glycemic goals may be appropriate for individual patients [36]

For CVD risk reduction in patients with diabetes, large benefits are seen when multiple risk factors are addressed globally. The American Diabetes Association recommends a BP less than 130/80 mmHg and suggests that the first-line therapy in diabetes should include an ACE inhibitor or angiotensin II receptor blocker. It is recommended that the lipid profile should be checked annually. In adults with low risk lipid values, the LDL cholesterol should be less than 100 mg/dL, HDL cholesterol >50 mg/dL, and triglycerides <150 mg/dL. Statin therapy should be added to lifestyle therapy, regardless of lipid levels for diabetic patients with overt CVD or without CVD who are over the age of 40 years and have one or more of other CVD risk factors. In individuals with overt CVD, the LDL goal is less than 70 mg/dL. Aspirin therapy as a primary prevention strategy in type 1 and type 2 should be considered in most men more than 50 and women more than 60 years of age who have at least one additional major risk factor. It is recommended to advise all diabetic patients not to smoke and include smoking cessation counseling and other forms of treatment as a component of diabetes care. Finally, regular exercise and a Mediterranean type diet are recommended.

Acknowledgement This work is supported by NIH R01-HL073101 and R01-HL107910 (JRS) and VA Merit Award (JRS).

References

1. Kannel WB, McGee DL. Diabetes and cardiovascular disease. The Framingham Study. J Am Med Assoc. 1979;241:2035–8.
2. Sowers JR, Whaley-Connell A, Hayden MR. The role of overweight and obesity in the cardiorenal syndrome. Cardiorenal Med. 2011;1:5–12.
3. Vlassara H, Bucala R, Striker L. Pathogenic effects of advanced glycosylation: biochemical, biologic and clinical implications for diabetes and aging. Lab Invest. 1994;70:138–51.
4. Bierhaus A, Hofmann MA, Ziegler R, et al. AGEs and their interaction with AGE-receptors in vascular disease and diabetes mellitus. I. The AGE concept. Cardiovasc Res. 1998;37: 586–600.

5. Koya D, King GL. Protein kinase C activation and the development of diabetes complications. Diabetes. 1998;47:859–66.
6. Vlassara H, Fuh H, Donnelly T, et al. Advanced glycation end products promote adhesion molecule (VCAM-1, ICAM-1) expression and atheroma formation in normal rabbits. Mol Med. 1995;1:447–56.
7. Egan BM, Lu G, Green EL. Vascular effects of non-esterified fatty acids: implications for the cardiovascular risk factor cluster. Prostaglandins Leukot Essent Fatty Acids. 1999;60:411–1406.
8. Toft I, Bonna KH, Ingebresten OC, et al. Fibrinolytic function after dietary supplementation with omega 3 polyunsaturated fatty acids. Arterioscler Thromb Vasc Biol. 1997;17:814–9.
9. Expert Panel on Detection, Evaluation, and Treatment of High Blood Cholesterol in Adults. Executive summary of the third report of the national cholesterol education program (NCEP) expert panel on detection, evaluation and treatment of high blood cholesterol in adults (Adult treatment panel III). J Am Med Assoc. 2001;285(19):2486–97. NIH Publication No. 01–3670, May 2001.
10. Figler RA, Wang Q, Srinivasan S, et al. Links between insulin resistance, adenosine A2B receptors, and inflammatory markers in mice and humans. Diabetes. 2011;60(2):669–79.
11. Yamauchi T, Kamon J, Waki H, et al. Fat derived hormone adiponectin reverses insulin resistance associated with both lipoatrophy and obesity. Nat Med. 2001;7:941–6.
12. Lau DC, Dhillon B, Yan H, et al. Adipokines: molecular links between obesity and atherosclerosis. Am J Physiol Heart Circ Physiol. 2005;288:H2031–41.
13. Ouchi N, Kihara S, Arita Y, et al. Novel modulator for endothelial adhesion molecules: adipocytes-derived plasma protein adiponectin. Circulation. 1999;100:2473–6.
14. O'Brien T, Nguyen TT, Zimmerman BR. Hyperlipidemia and diabetes mellitus. Mayo Clin Proc. 1998;73:969–76.
15. Schimdt AM, Hori O, Brett J, et al. Cellular receptors for advanced glycation end products: implications for induction of oxidant stress and cellular dysfunction in the pathogenesis of vascular lesion. Arterioscler Thromb. 1994;14:1521–8.
16. Ross R. Atherosclerosis: an inflammatory disease. N Engl J Med. 1999;340:115–26.
17. Szalai AJ, Van Ginkel FW, Wang Y, et al. Complement-dependent acute phase expression of C-reactive protein and serum amyloid P-component. J Immunol. 2000;165:1030–5.
18. Schneider DJ, Sobel BE. Diabetes and thrombosis. In: Johnstone MT, Veves A, editors. Diabetes and cardiovascular disease. Totowa, NJ: Humana Press; 2001. p. 107–28.
19. Cardillo C, Nambi SS, Kilcoyne CM, et al. Insulin stimulates both endothelium and nitric oxide activity in the human forearm. Circulation. 1999;100:820–5.
20. Cooper SA, Whaley-Connell A, Habibi J, et al. Renin-angiotensin-aldosterone system and oxidative stress in cardiovascular insulin resistance. Am J Physiol Heart Circ Physiol. 2007;293:H2009–23.
21. Ren J, Pulakat L, Whaley-Connell A, et al. Mitochondrial biogenesis in the metabolic syndrome and cardiovascular disease. J Mol Med. 2010;88:993–1001.
22. Lowell BB, Shulman GI. Mitochondrial dysfunction and type 2 diabetes. Science. 2005;307:384–7.
23. Whaley-Connell A, Pulakat L, DeMarco VG, et al. Overnutrition and the cardiorenal syndrome: use of a rodent model to examine mechanisms. Cardiorenal Med. 2011;1:23–30.
24. Intensive blood-glucose control with sulphonylureas or insulin compared with conventional treatment and risk of complications in patients with type 2 diabetes (UKPDS33). UK Prospective Diabetes Study (UKPDS) Group. Lancet. 1998;352:837–853.
25. Diabetes Control and Complications Trial Research Group. The effect of intensive treatment of diabetes on the development and progression of long-term complications in insulin-dependent diabetes mellitus. N EnglJMed. 1993;329:977–86.
26. Gaede P, Vedel P, Larsren N, et al. Multifactorial intervention and cardiovascular disease in patients with type 2 diabetes. N Engl J Med. 2003;348:383–90.
27. Del Prato S. Megatrials in type 2 Diabetes. From excitement to frustration? Diabetologia. 2009;52:1219–26.

28. Duckworth W, Abraira C, Moritz T, et al. Glucose control and vascular complications in veterans with type 2 diabetes. N Engl J Med. 2009;369:129–40.
29. Heller SR, ADVANCE Collaborative Group. A summary of the ADVANCE Trial. Diabetes Care. 2009;32 Suppl 2:S357–62.
30. The Action to Control Cardiovascular Risk in Diabetes Study Group. Effects of intensive glucose lowering in type 2 diabetes. N Engl J Med. 2008;358:2545–59.
31. Dale AC, Vatten LJ, Nilsen TI, et al. Secular decline in mortality from coronary heart disease in adults with diabetes mellitus: cohort study. Br Med J. 2008;337:99–102.
32. The Diabetes Control and Complications Trial/Epidemiology of Diabetes Interventions and Complications (DCCT/EDIC) Study Research Group. Intensive diabetes treatment and cardiovascular disease in patients with type 1 diabetes. N Engl J Med. 2005;353:2643–53.
33. Holman RR, Paul SK, Bethel MA, et al. 10-Year follow-up of intensive glucose control in type 2 diabetes. N Engl J Med. 2008;359:1577–89.
34. Gerstein HC, Miller ME, Byington RP, et al. Effects of intensive glucose lowering in type 2 diabetes. N Engl J Med. 2008;358:580–91.
35. Ray KK, Seshasai SR, Wijesuriya S, et al. Effect of intensive control of glucose on cardiovascular outcomes and death in patients with diabetes mellitus: a meta-analysis of randomized controlled trials. Lancet. 2009;373:1765–72.
36. American Diabetes Association. Standards of medical care in diabetes—2010. Diabetes Care. 2010;33:S11–48.

Chapter 8
Hypertension, Diabetes, and the Eye

Douglas R. Lazzaro and Eric Shrier

Hypertensive Retinopathy

Hypertension or high blood pressure remains a serious problem not only here in the USA but worldwide as well. In the USA, almost one in three adults are afflicted with high blood pressure [1] while in Europe, it is the leading cause of long-term medical care [2]. There are varied incidences of hypertension in country with some areas having up to 50% of the chronically treated population being treated for this condition.

Hypertension affects males and females to a similar extent and its incidence increases with age. African Americans in the USA have a higher incidence of disease, and the severity of disease in all groups can have an impact on end-organ damage.

The sequelae of hypertension include stroke, cardiac disease, renal disease, and loss of vision to name but a few. Hypertension affecting the eye is known as hypertensive retinopathy and can cause vision loss in a number of ways. The first description of this entity dates back to 1892 by Gunn [3]. Its more recent classifications have been described previously [4, 5] (see Fig. 8.1).

D.R. Lazzaro, M.D., F.A.C.S., F.A.A.O. (✉)
Department of Ophthalmology, The Richard C. Troutman, M.D. Distinguished Chair
in Ophthalmology and Ophthalmic Microsurgery, SUNY Downstate Medical Center,
Brooklyn, NY 11203, USA

UHB, SUNY Downstate Medical Center, Brooklyn, NY 11203, USA

KCHC, HHC, Brooklyn, NY 11203, USA

LICH, SUNY Downstate Medical Center, Brooklyn, NY 11203, USA
e-mail: Douglas.lazzaro@downstate.edu

E. Shrier, M.D.
Department of Ophthalmology, SUNY Downstate Medical Center, Brooklyn, NY 11203, USA

S.I. McFarlane and G.L. Bakris (eds.), *Diabetes and Hypertension: Evaluation
and Management*, Contemporary Diabetes, DOI 10.1007/978-1-60327-357-2_8,
© Springer Science+Business Media New York 2012

Keith-Wagener-Barker classification of hypertensive retinopathy:

Group I- Minimal constriction of the retinal arterioles with some tortuosity in patients with mild HTN

Group II- Retinal abnormalities include those of group I, with more definite focal narrowing and arteriolovenous nicking in patients with minimal or no other systemic involvement

Group III- Abnormalities include those in groups I, II and also hemorrhages and exudates and vasospastic changes that include focal arteriolar constriction and cotton-wool spots. Many of these patients have identifiable cardiac, cerebral, or renal dysfunction.

Group IV- Above abnormalities are present and more severe plus optic disc edema. Elschning's spots are present in some. The cardiac, cerebral and renal diseases are more severe,

Fig. 8.1 Keith–Wagener–Barker classification of hypertensive retinopathy

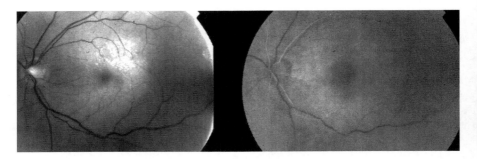

Fig. 8.2 Red-free (*left image*) and early transit fluorescein angiographic image (set *right*) of a left eye depicting retinal arteriolar attenuation (arteriole fluoresces white in this early transit frame of the angiogram)

Hypertensive retinopathy is most commonly a bilateral disease although rarely it can present unilaterally. Hypertensive retinopathy occurs in men and women, yet in one European study looking at Afro-Caribbeans and Europeans aged 40–64, a higher prevalence of retinopathy was seen in the Afro-Caribbean group compared to Europeans and also women when compared to men [6]. Smoking increases the risk of hypertensive retinopathy, and the disease can be seen concomitantly with diabetic retinopathy.

Hypertensive retinopathy and its clinical picture can be seen as a direct result of the pathological changes taking place in the vascular system [7]. Increased tone of the arteriolar system leads to narrowing seen by the ophthalmoscope. Indeed, the ratio of venule diameter to arteriole diameter increases as disease progresses. Subsequent damage to the arteriolar wall leads to silver or copper wiring seen by the physician. Arteriovenular crossing (nicking) changes take place as the arteriolar wall stiffens leading in some cases to venular obstruction, which will be further mentioned later in the discussion (see Figs. 8.2 and 8.3).

Fig. 8.3 *Color image*
shows severe hypertensive
retinopathy with the
appearance of an
"impending" central retinal
vein occlusion. *Arrow* depicts
severe A–V nicking

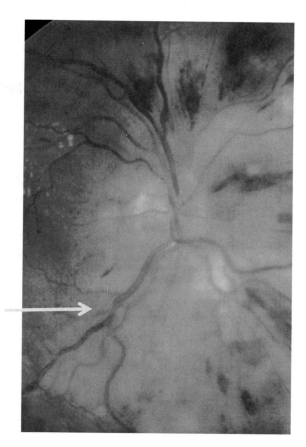

Incompetence of the arteriolar system can also lead to vascular leakage of lipid seen as hard exudates and hemorrhage most often seen in the nerve fiber layer. The lipid can be seen as ring shaped or as a macular star (see Fig. 8.4). Infarcts of the nerve fiber layer by ischemic vasculature can lead to cotton wool spots, a telltale sign of impaired circulation when seen in conjunction with hypertension. The cotton wool spots (see Fig. 8.5) are often referred to as soft exudates, a misnomer as they represent an infarct and not an exudate. It should be kept in mind that numerous other causes of nerve fiber layer infarcts exist, but taken in their totality with other historical and physical findings can be ascribed to a high blood pressure abnormality in the right clinical setting.

The loss of vision in hypertension can be a direct result of the disease or a secondary phenomenon. Clearly, the patient who develops fluid leakage into the macular area where exquisite function is needed for perfect vision will suffer temporary or permanent loss of vision. The patient who develops ischemia to the macula (ischemic maculopathy) likewise may show impairment of vision, often irreversible. The development of stage 4 hypertensive retinopathy with optic nerve edema

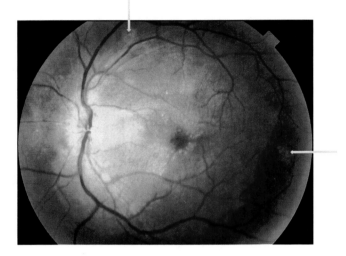

Fig. 8.4 Color fundus photo of a *left eye* depicting "Macular star" formation and optic nerve edema. There is arteriolar attenuation and venous dilatation. *Arrows* indicate early "Elschnig spots"

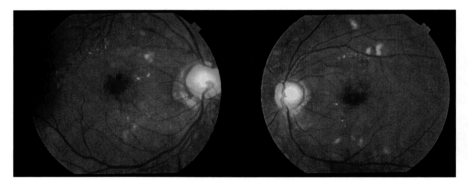

Fig. 8.5 Color fundus photos of *right* and *left eyes*. Severe nonproliferative diabetic retinopathy and coincident hypertension have resulted in bilateral diabetic macular edema. Multiple bilateral cotton-wool spots representing nerve fiber layer infarcts are seen

(see Fig. 8.6) can have serious long lasting implications for vision. An optic nerve compromised by poor circulation will develop atrophy if left untreated [8]. Bilateral, exudative retinal detachment may occur with a precipitous rise in blood pressure (see Fig. 8.7). This condition is marked by "shifting" sub-retinal fluid, located inferiorly, due to the effects of gravity.

Retinal arteriole macroaneurysms (see Fig. 8.8) can also be associated with hypertension in the majority of cases [9, 10]. A weakened histologically altered aged blood vessel can dilate under the influence leading to the aneurysm. The dilated abnormal area can then rupture leading to retinal hemorrhage.

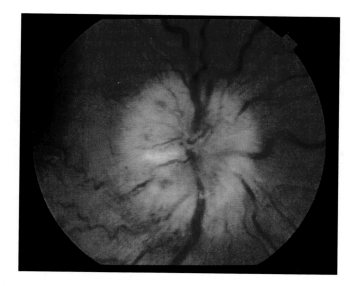

Fig. 8.6 Color photo of a *right eye* depicting optic nerve edema and macular edema. Enlargement of the nerve shown to the *right*. Blurring of the disc margins and obscuration of the tiny capillaries as they cross the margins signify "true" disc edema

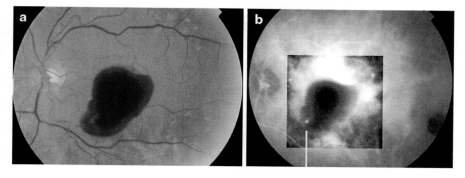

Fig. 8.7 (**a**) Bilateral, inferior exudative retinal detachment in a patient with hypertensive emergency. (**b**) Resolution of retinal detachment after normotensive status achieved. (*Arrow*) An early Elschnig spot is seen representing area of choroidal infarct

Hypertension can affect the choroid which appears sensitive to pathologic altera-tions [11]. A number of fundus lesions can be seen including the Elschnig spot and the Seigrist streak.

Hypertension can be a risk factor for both retinal artery and retinal vein occlusive disease [12]. An occlusion of a branch (see Fig. 8.9) or central retinal vein (see Fig. 8.10) can be accompanied by mild to severe vision impairment. Artery occlu-sions in the retina also have hypertension as a major risk factor and the central reti-nal artery type (see Fig. 8.11) leads in essentially all patients to a complete loss of

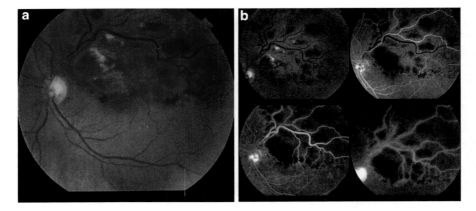

Fig. 8.8 (a) Retinal arteriolar macroaneurysm suspected in color photo of a *left eye*. (b) Highlighted early frame indocyanine-green (ICG) angiogram: the lesion (*arrow*) was blocked by a large secondary pre-retinal hemorrhage, necessitating ICG imaging for diagnosis and localization. The legion was treated with thermal laser ablation

Fig. 8.9 Left color fundus photo depicting the late sequelae of a central retinal artery occlusion. Optic nerve shows pallor, and ghost vessels are evident. Circular, black "Elschnig spots" are seen, representing localized choroidal infarctions. There is pigment mottling in the macular area. Vision is bare light perception (LP)

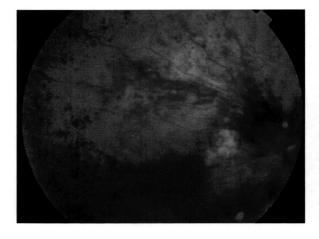

Fig. 8.10 Fundus photo of a *right eye* with central retinal vein occlusion

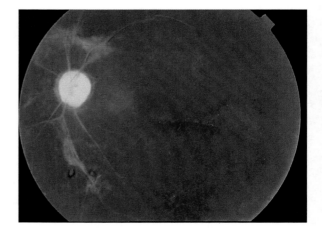

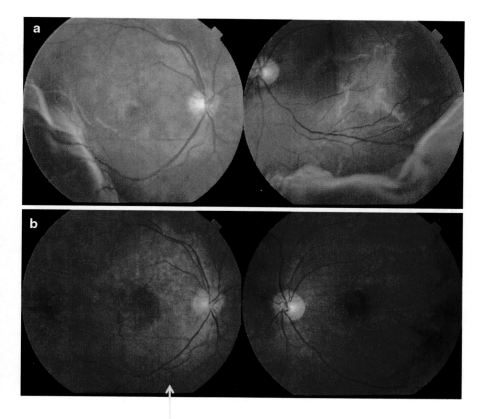

Fig. 8.11 (**a**) Color fundus photo of a left eye depicting branch retinal vein occlusion. (**b**) Fluorescein angiographic image series showing hypo fl uorescence due to ischemia and blockage by intraretinal blood. There is late staining of the veins in the late frame (lower right)

central vision [13]. Whereas central retinal artery occlusions occur mostly due to thrombus formation, branch retinal artery occlusions more commonly occur from embolic phenomena.

There is an association of hypertensive retinopathy and stroke. Evidence suggests that the presence of retinopathy may have an association with cerebrovascular disease [14] and with different types of cerebrovascular events [15]. An extensive prospective study of patients with acute lacunar infarcts showed a correlation with a number of factors in the retinal microvasculature [16]. A prospective study looking at ischemic stroke patients within 1 week of the event demonstrated that there was a higher rate of recurrent cerebrovascular events in patients that had either retinal focal arteriolar narrowing or AV nicking [17]. Another recent study has shown that hypertensive retinopathic abnormalities related to stroke can allow clinicians to further individualize a risk profile for stroke to each patient and potentially guide treatment strategies [18].

Anterior ischemic optic neuropathy of the non-arteritic type has hypertension as a risk factor as well [19, 20]. This type of optic nerve infarction tends to have a better visual prognosis than when caused by temporal arteritis but still can have permanent visual deterioration.

Important and relevant to this entire section is the need to control high blood pressure in all of these manifestations in the eye. The retina is being affected as are other end organs in these settings. The normalization of blood pressure in our patients afflicted with this disease can no doubt reduce the incidence of ophthalmic dysfunction.

Diabetes and the Eye

Diabetes is the leading cause of new blindness in the USA among adults aged 20–74 [21]. Given its propensity to affect relatively young adults in the prime of their working lives', with long duration of expected survival, the economic and social cost to our society is terribly high. A known or recently diagnosed diabetic patient who complains of visual distortion, "blurry vision," or "floaters" must be taken very seriously, as it may herald the development of what may be or become irreversible blindness. Furthermore, diabetic eye disease is closely associated with other serious end-organ damage (i.e., chronic renal insufficiency, peripheral neuropathy, and coronary artery disease) [22].

Anterior Segment Manifestations

Autonomic neuropathy resulting from chronic hyperglycemia may affect the corneal sensation (CN V) thereby reducing the necessary compensatory production of the aqueous component of tears, reducing the efficacy of the tear-film as it bathes the cornea. This may manifest as a complaint of eye fatigue such as that occurs with prolonged reading, foreign-body sensation due to "dry eyes (syndrome)," punctate epithelial keratitis (tiny erosions), or keratitis sicca (very dry eyes). Treatment is aimed at replacement of the aqueous component of tears (i.e., artificial tears, q.i.d or PRN) or in more advanced cases with gel lubricants (i.e., puralube) or topical cyclosporine A (Restasis) b.i.d. More recalcitrant cases may be treated by punctual occlusion with silicone punctual plugs.

Refractive changes in the status of the human crystalline human lens is well known to occur with precipitous changes in serum glycemic status. Blurred vision is in fact a common presenting symptom of Type 1 diabetes. Visual disturbance certainly occurs due to osmotic changes in the lens itself; hyperglycemia induces swelling and "fattening" of the lens altering its power, which induces a myopic or "near-sighted" shift in lens refractive power. The characteristics of the particular visual disturbance depends upon the patient's native refractive state. In emmetropic (normal) or myopic (near-sighted) persons, distance vision may be preferentially worsened, while near vision may in fact be unchanged. Three to four months of tight glycemic control usually results in refractive shift back to the native state. A temporary change in eyeglass prescription may be needed during this period.

Osmotic changes may affect the nucleus and cortex of the lens in a temporary or permanent fashion, resulting in oxidative damage to lens constituents (a and b crystalline proteins). The "Classic" changes to the crystalline lens which occurs over a longer period of time involves the posterior capsule of the lens [posterior subcapsular cataract (PSC)]. In the setting of long-standing, poorly controlled diabetes, PSC is not usually reversible. Cataract which persists after 3–4 months of "fairly good" glycemic control (i.e., FBS <200) are treated by cataract extraction and intraocular lens implantation if a new eyeglass or contact-lens prescription is not visually satisfactory. A notable exception to conservative management is where the lens changes are so significant so as to impede the view of the fundus and hence necessary evaluation and/or treatment of diabetic retinopathy.

Persons with longstanding diabetes usually experience accelerated presbyopia, which is the inability to read at the normal reading distance (at about 14 in.) without an optical reading addition to their eyeglass prescription. Persons who are hyperopic (far-sighted) will require a reading addition to their prescription earlier than the myopic (near-sighted) individuals. Accelerated presbyopia is felt to be due to reduced accommodative amplitudes of the ciliary body secondary to autonomic neuropathy affecting CN III. Perhaps there could be some contribution due to the premature "hardening" of the crystalline lens due to hyperglycemia (crystalline lens proteins alpha- and beta-crystallins are oxidized). This clinically manifests as an increased near-prescription requirement between the ages of 50 and 75.

Double vision (diplopia) that is associated with diabetes may result from significant posterior subcapsular cataract (PSC) formation (subacute or chronic),or from true strabismus [an esotropia inward (CN VI) or exotropia outward (CN III) eye muscle deviation of one eye]. Longstanding diabetes occasionally results in acute neuro-paresis (eye deviated in with CN VI or eye deviated out in CN III palsy). This is yet another example of an eye manifestation from autonomic neuropathy. To be attributable merely to diabetes, though, ophthalmic and neurologic consultation should be urgently obtained. The differential diagnosis of recent onset exotropia (deviation of eyes outward) includes consideration of an anterior communicating artery macroaneurysm of the brain (compressing CN III), which can lead to massive-subarachnoid hemorrhagic stroke and death if undiagnosed.

Interestingly, headache and eye pain may be associated with either condition. The autonomic neuropathy in this instance is microvascular in nature and is potentiated by systemic hypertension. Importantly, the nerve fibers subserving constriction of the pupil of the iris are spared in diabetic CN III paresis, where they are affected in aneurysmal-associated CN III exo-deviations, resulting in a dilated "blown" pupil.

Diabetes associated strabismus usually resolves fully over the course of weeks or months.

The iris may become involved in long-standing diabetes. The iris stroma may become atrophic in lightly pigmented individuals with blue eyes (so-called, histopathologic lacy vacuolization) or in advanced diabetic eye disease due to rubeosis iridis (Ruby red eye in Latin).

Neovascular glaucoma (NVG) is a devastating eye disease, since it results in a blind and painful eye. It most often occurs in the setting of severely ischemic Proliferative retinopathy, but may arise in association with other retinal vascular conditions. NVG occurs when neovascularization of the anterior chamber angle occurs. The "angle" is where aqueous humor produced by the ciliary body drains from the eye. Outflow is impeded as the neovascularization fibroses and closes the anatomical angle. The process may be reversed with aggressive treatment if part of the angle remains open.

Posterior Eye Involvement

Diabetes affects the capillary network of the retinal vascular circulation preferentially. Interestingly, the deeper choroid and choriocapillaris are not typically affected, perhaps since these vessels are fenestrated and dissimilar to the capillaries of the inner retina. Significant and permanent vision loss that results from diabetes is always due to posterior-segment ocular involvement until proven otherwise. Vision loss due to retinal problems may become irreparable with a short passage of time (weeks or months). Impending, permanent visual loss due to retinal problems should be always considered in those patients who you see with possible and known diabetes, unless it can be proven otherwise. It is important to note that the occasional patient goes permanently blind from diabetic retinopathy even when well controlled.

Visual loss in diabetic retinopathy is best classified as moderate [doubling of the visual angle (i.e., 20/20 to 20/40) or severe (worse than 20/200)]. The goal of treatment in diabetic retinopathy is to lessen the chance of vision loss, be it moderate vision loss in the case of macular edema or severe vision loss in proliferative diabetic retinopathy (PDR).

Highly threatening retinopathy in the setting of diabetes is usually due to PDR, and it often presents in the very advanced stages. Given the anatomical posterior ocular location of the retina, it may not be apparent or visible to the patient or to the primary-care doctor.

Advanced means of examination (i.e., indirect ophthalmoscopy and slit-lamp biomicroscopy) are required to appreciate the condition. It cannot be inexpertly differentiated from the reversible aforementioned causes of vision loss (i.e., refractive error or cataract), and the extent can be often missed in the care of the inexperienced examiner (see Fig. 8.12). Duration and severity of the systemic disease is not at all a reliable factor in differentiating permanent, severe eye disease from that which is treatable and temporary; each case must be looked at individually.

Permanent sight-threatening eye disease involving the retina can and does exist in the setting of the, "I don't even have diabetes" patient. Previously undiscovered genetic factors governing retinal vascular perfusion and formation of neovascularization may explain this occurrence. Patients have gone blind from mild and late-treated Type II DM and then soon thereafter develop chronic renal failure (CRF) and a need for urgent hemodialysis.

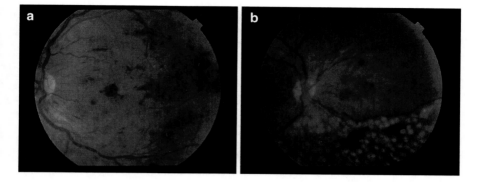

Fig. 8.12 (**a**) This color fundus photo of the *left eye* depicts a 24-year-old man with fairly good visual acuity (20/30). A casual observer might say that he had diabetic retinopathy, with "some dot-blot heme." In fact, he has very severe proliferative retinopathy, with NVD and diffuse macular edema. The conspicuous absence of lipid, bleeding and fibrosis make correct recognition difficult at first glance. (**b**) Photo of the same eye later that day after PRP was applied. He opted to be initially treated with simultaneous injection of intravitreal steroids

Annual screening eye exams are of great value, assuming they are provided by a qualified eye care physician. Given the great importance of vision and the impact of early treatment, patients require close lifelong observation by a qualified doctor (at least twice per annum when diabetic retinopathy is diagnosed). True IDDM can be seen initially at 5 years from diagnosis, and others should be seen soon after diagnosis.

Nonproliferative diabetic retinopathy (NPDR) is classified as mild ("background") (see Fig. 8.13) moderate (see Fig. 8.14) and severe ("pre-proliferative"). It necessarily predates PDR, but is variable in its manifestations and significance on vision. Often reassurance and observation are all that is necessary. But its extent is sometimes underestimated. If patients come under good glycemic and hypertension control, anatomical and visual prognoses are fairly good. Retinal disease may actually paradoxically worsen though after glycemic, blood-pressure, and serum lipid indices are optimized [22].

Diabetic retinopathy is caused by retinal vascular abnormalities closely akin to that which occurs in the renal glomeruli. The pathogenesis and pathophysiology are probably identical. The accepted theory involves hyperglycemia induced basement membrane thickening, loss of pericytes, and endothelial dysfunction. Hypoxia, oxidative stress, inflammation, and protein damage causes vascular endothelial growth factor (VEGF) to be upregulated. Substantive changes in native blood vessels (see Fig. 8.15) occur during the early stages (nonproliferative or "background" diabetic retinopathy), seen as microaneurysmal saccular changes in capillaries and small intraretinal "dot-blot" hemorrhages [23]. Cotton-wool spots, signifying nerve-fiber layer ischemia and infarct are also seen but are not pathogneumonic changes of diabetes, as they are commonly seen to result from hypertension and collagen-vascular diseases.

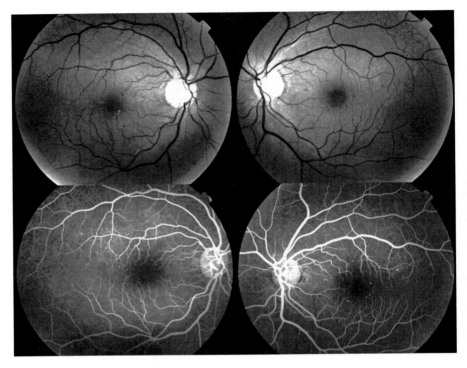

Fig. 8.13 Red-free (*top*) and mid-phase fluorescein angiographic images (*bottom*) depict microaneurysms — seen as hyperfluorescent spots. A small amount of lipid is seen inferior to the foveola *top right* image, indicating CSDME. This would be monitored closely, and patient would be advised of the great importance of HTN, BS and lipid control

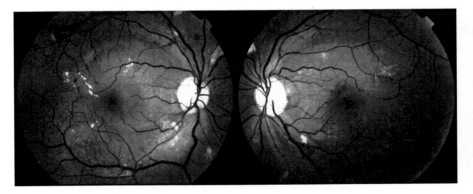

Fig. 8.14 *Right* (**a**) and *left* (**b**) eye red-free photos depicting moderate NPDR and bilateral CSDME. Lipid is threatening the foveal center (**a**), and a peri-foveal microaneurysm is causing foveal edema (**b**). Both eyes display cotton-wool spots indicative of moderate nonproliferative diabetic retinopathy. Patient was treated with focal laser (**a**) and intravitreal therapy (**b**), as the microvascular abnormality was judged too close to the fovea to treat safely with laser. Both eyes must be monitored very closely for progression to PDR. PRP laser may be necessary within months, or if patient is judged unreliable to follow-up

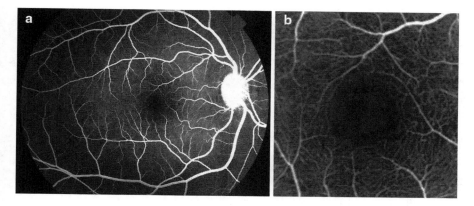

Fig. 8.15 (a) This is a normal fundus fluorescein mid-phase circulation image of the *right eye*. The retinal vessels show fluorescence about 1 min after fluorescein intravenous dye injection. (b) Note the healthy (magnified) appearance of the capillary network surrounding the anatomical foveola. The extent of the central black area represents the so-called foveolar avascular zone

Preproliferative retinopathy that is seen just prior to the proliferative type includes compensatory vascular anomalies due to VEGF, such as intraretinal microvascular abnormalities (IRMA), venous beading, and extensive capillary nonperfusion.

Retinal changes tend to be chronic and go largely unnoticed for years, as they almost never cause visual abnormalities. As areas of retinal ischemia broaden, more VEGF and inflammatory mediators are poured into the vitreous which impacts the native, but dysfunctional retinal capillaries. Leakage occurs into the retina, which comes to exceed the resorptive capacity of the blood vessels and the underlying retinal pigment epithelial cells.

Lipid falls out of fluid suspension when fluid is reabsorbed. Thickening and lipid deposition are included in the grading scheme of clinically significant diabetic macular edema (CSDME). Vision can be normal and the condition may go unnoticed. Visual acuity is not even part of the classification scheme. Retinal thickening and lipid which comes to affect the macula eventually causes moderate visual change, however. Late stage severe or untreated disease often results in severe vision loss, "legal blindness."

Overexpression of VEGF causes the formation of new abnormal blood vessels, in their attempt to recapitulate the architecture of the retinal capillary network. They are always pathological, however, and usually lead to bleeding and distortion of the retina with concomitant severe vision loss. They are seen to proliferate behind the vitreous body on the surface of the optic disc and retina as tiny, fragile capillaries, "neovascularization of the disc" (NVD) and "neovascularization elsewhere" (NVE) (see Figs. 8.16 and 8.17). Bleeding emanates from the incompetent vessels. This may occur spontaneously, especially in the case of uncontrolled hypertension, or as a result of vitreous traction. Tractional retinal detachment (TRD) occurs as a

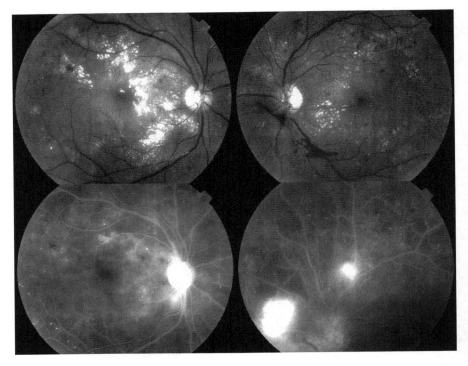

Fig. 8.16 Red-free photos (*top*) and late-phase fluorescein angiographic photos (*bottom*) of the *right* and *left* eyes. Diffuse CSDME with circinate lipid exuation is evident

result of involution of neovascularization fibrovascular tissue (see Fig. 8.18), as it is constantly pulled upon by the vitreous body. Eventual separation of the vitreous from the optic nerve and retina, where it is firmly attached embryologically, may also induce bleeding, TRD, and retinal breaks.

Vitreous separation tends to occur later in diabetics, owing to alteration in their constituent proteins as it is stickier than usual. Abnormal splitting and lamination of the vitreous body is seen at the time of vitreous surgery as well. Vitreous that fails to separate from the macula proper is thought to possibly contribute to macular edema, and can itself distort the foveal pit, the so-called vitreo-macular traction syndrome (VMTS) which is best treated by surgical release, pars-plana vitrectomy (PPV).

Three-port PPV is commonly performed in the setting of diabetes. Indications for PPV in the diabetic may include aforementioned significant cases of VMTS, or when macular distortion occurs by contractile fibrovascular tissue (see Fig. 8.18); non-clearing and significant vitreous hemorrhage; TRD involving the macula, and complex retinal detachments with open retinal breaks. Modern PPV is seen as faster and safer than when it was in its infancy (1970s–1990s), so its use and indications have expanded somewhat.

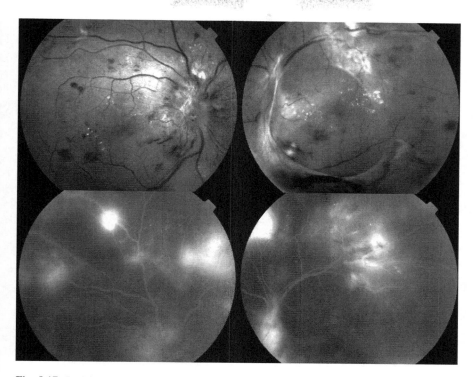

Fig. 8.17 Red-free photos (*top*) and late-circulation fluorescein angiographic images (*bottom*). Large areas of hypofluorescence are seen consistent with nonperfusion/ischemia. Neovascularization, which is hyperfluorescent, tends to occur at borders of these areas (so-called watershed zones). Fibrosis is evident in the *upper right* photo, in a commonly seen configuration. This is very severe PDR of both eyes (o.u.)

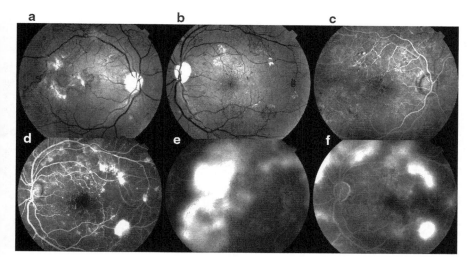

Fig. 8.18 (**a–f**) This 45-year-old long-standing IDDM patient has very severe, flat NVE (**a, b**) which has invaded the macula in the *right eye* (**a**). He recently had PRP at another facility in the o.d. (**a, c**) and attributes his 20/25 vision to that event. Extensive hyperfluorescent areas represent NVE (**d–f**). There is a conspicuous absence of NVD and VH, though, and his uncorrected vision is excellent (20/25R and 20/20L). He is at high risk of sudden, near simultaneous blindness. His macular disease will be treated with intravitreal therapy (Avastin) *R*, focal and grid laser *L*, and aggressive scatter PRP laser (o.u.)

Instruments range in size from 20 to 23 to 25-gage. Only the former gauge requires sutures. Removal of the vitreous body's posterior hyaloid membrane and most of the vitreous body substance removes the "scaffold" implicated in formation of TRD, VMTS and recurrent vitreous hemorrhage. It is not without significant risks, i.e., re-bleeding (10–20%), infection rarely, macular hole, glaucoma, or optic neuropathy which can result in permanent vision loss. Persons who were previously untreated with laser PRP may do especially poorly. In the earlier days of vitreo-retinal surgery, PPV for PDR carried high risks, about a 10% chance of severe and permanent blindness (NLP vision) [24].

Intravitreal anti-VEGF agents are now used extensively for PDR preoperatively in cases where profuse neovascularization exists. Caution must be exercised though, as involution and contraction of neovascular vessels occurs very rapidly and this may induce progressive TRD, retinal breaks, and complex retinal detachment.

The treatment of CSDME based on results of the early treatment of diabetic retinopathy study (ETDRS) is focal laser treatment. It can reduce the chance of suffering moderate vision loss by about 50% over several years [25, 26]. Focal laser entails applying small spots of thermal laser under direct visualization to leaky microaneurysms which are visible at the slit-lamp and further localized on intravenous fluorescein angiography (IVFA) (see Fig. 8.13). IVFA is very helpful in identifying areas of peripheral retinal nonperfusion and cases with coexisting macular ischemia. Historically, a grid-like pattern of laser was applied in cases of diffuse macular edema, but this is now performed less frequently. Judicious focal laser is still the "gold standard" treatment for CSDME and very useful in cases of discrete CSDME when microaneurysms are not foveal involving.

Focal laser is less useful in cases with diffuse macular edema (see Fig. 8.16) and cases where microaneurysms are located within the foveal avascular zone. Any type of diabetic macular edema which is refractory to repeated focal laser is offered in conjunction with anti-VEGF intravitreal therapy [bevacizumab (Avastin) or ranibizumab (Lucentis)]. Laser treatment is offered based on results of the ETDRS, respective of significant macular thickening with or without lipid presence threatening the foveal center [25, 26]. Anti-VEGF intravitreal treatment is highly effective, as VEGF is strongly implicated in vascular leakage from the abnormal diabetic capillaries [27, 28]. The duration of action is a short 1–2 months, so monotherapy with anti-VEGF offers a temporary benefit, thus being less advantageous than focal laser treatment.

Alternative treatments include intravitreal steroid injection, which carries the high risk of ocular hypertension with possible glaucoma and cataract. Effects on the retina are quite transitory and tachyphylaxis is often seen. Specially formulated intravitreal steroids [i.e., sustained-release dexamethasone (Ozurdex)] are a favored treatment in chronic edema cases especially where lipid has precipitated and deposited near the foveal center. Focal laser induces long-term durable benefit versus intravitreal steroids [29].

PPV with or without internal limited-membrane peeling is a last ditch option for treatment of severe diffuse CSDME. The therapeutic response to the aforementioned modalities are best followed with serial ocular coherence tomography (OCT)

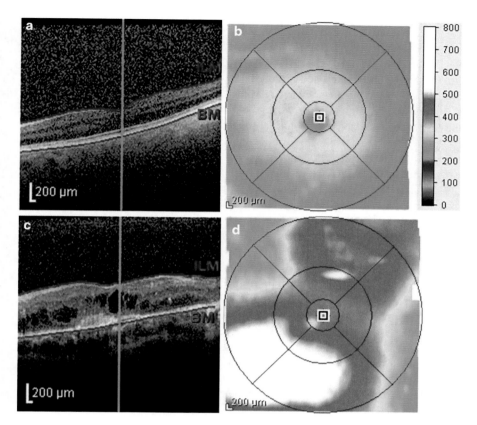

Fig. 8.19 Upper images depict SD-OCT (Heidelberg) (*left*) in a normal macula and its associated topographic thickness map in microns (*right*). Lower images depict SD-OCT (*left*) in chronic CSDME and associated topographic thickness map in microns (*right*). *ILM* internal limiting membrane, *BM* Bruch's membrane

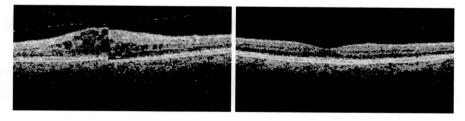

Fig. 8.20 SD-OCT image (Optovue™) which depict macular edema of the *right eye* (**a**) and a nice foveal contour several months after focal laser of the *left* (**b**)

(see Figs. 8.19 and 8.20) and IVFA. Spectral domain high resolution OCT is a great advance as it provides noncontact, quantification of therapeutic response in the macula noting, however, that IVFA is still needed to assess the retinal circulation.

The treatment of PDR is based on results of the diabetic retinopathy study (DRS). Pan-retinal photocoagulation (PRP) is beneficial in reducing the chance of severe vision loss over several years time [30, 31]. Consideration of the presence, location (on the disc or elsewhere), and extent of neovascularization along with the presence or absence of vitreous hemorrhage are made to determine if laser is appropriate. In this practical algorithm, derived from the results of the DRS, neovascualrization of the disc which is extensive should be treated with PRP, while NVE must be more profuse or be associated with vitreous hemorrhage to warrant treatment. Patients who are judged to be at high risk of progression or non-compliant are usually offered earlier treatment. In PRP, large 300–500 μm spots of laser are applied under direct visualization to the peripheral retina. This is done to basically "kill off" the dying, ischemic peripheral retina, which is implicated in pathologic VEGF release. Reduction of VEGF causes a reduction in stimulating neovascularization and macular edema formation. Furthermore, PRP laser treatment "tacks down" the neurosensory retina to the underlying retinal pigment epithelium (RPE), which at least in theory lessens the chance that it will detach.

PRP laser treatment is still the "gold standard" for PDR, as it is very safe, effective, and very durable in its impact. PRP, when indicated, is ordinarily supplied in aliquots of 650–2,500 spots as tolerated (see Fig. 8.12). Higher amounts of laser may predispose the patient (and treating doctor) to significant discomfort and inflammation. Topical anesthesia (Tetracaine 1%) is sufficient to allow laser treatment in the office setting. Peri-bulbar infiltration with an injection of lidocaine 1% may be provided, although significant periorbital swelling and risks of permanent vision loss from the injection itself must be considered. Mentally challenged, emotionally unstable or disturbed individuals may be treated in the operating room or ambulatory surgery-center setting under monitored anesthesia.

It bears mentioning that PDR often causes severe and permanent vision loss. As the disease is somewhat unpredictable, the patient must be advised of the great importance of timely and consistent follow-up. A fully functional, active, employed, driving adult can go bilaterally blind in weeks to months (Fig. 8.21). Macular ischemia resulting from expansion of the normal foveolar avascular zone may occur in uncontrolled diabetes with hypertension and causes irreversible, severe vision loss. Its temporal occurrence is unpredictable.

In the setting of significant diabetic vitreous hemorrhage in PDR, properly applied PRP laser is always very helpful, as it directly reduces the load of VEGF delivered to the functioning retina. It makes a surgical cure more likely if deemed necessary. In the diabetic patient with minimal prior laser, or where significant laser cannot be safely applied through the vitreous hemorrhage, proximate treatment with vitrectomy is usually indicated [24]. If the status of the retina cannot be determined or confirmed with B-scan ultrasound exam, proximate surgery is indicated. Some laser can ordinarily be applied in a significant fashion by the retinal specialist. If laser has been previously applied in a modest fashion, and vitreous floaters/blurry vision is not due to a retinal detachment, observation is indicated. The patient is

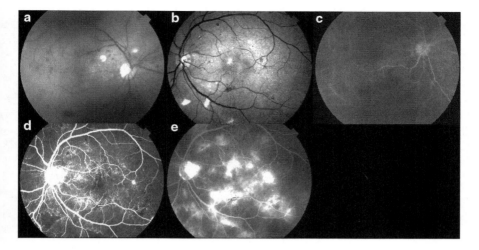

Fig. 8.21 This patient had "perfect" vision until occurrence of "floaters" *R* several days prior to presentation. He had severe PDR which was occult and unrecognized until she experienced a "sentinel bleed" in the form of VH R (**a**, **c**). Aggressive PRP will be applied in an exigent fashion, as further bleeding will necessitate urgent PPV. *L* will be treated with aggressive PRP (**b**, **d**, **e**). Surgery in this setting is quite treacherous as the risk of intra- and postoperative bleeding is high in the un- or inadequately lasered eye

followed at monthly intervals. Fill-in PRP is applied to untreated retinal areas until hemorrhage subsides and neovascularization begins to regress. Until that time, the patient is instructed to sleep with the head of the bed elevated at 30° (on two-pillows) to potentiate gravitational inferior settling of the hemorrhage.

Even with sufficient laser (4,000–6,000 PRP total laser spots), rebleeding into the vitreous may occur though due to vitreous traction on persistent neovascular tissue. Vitreous opacities may persist indefinitely to some extent. Patients treated with indicated significant laser treatment early on in the course of the disease do quite well and usually maintain vision that will allow important life activities such as driving and reading to continue. Severe bilateral vision loss represents an 85% loss of body function. There is a strong benefit from strict control of diabetes, HTN, and abnormal lipids [22]. For most patients who benefit from aggressive screening and treatment, vision loss may be reversed with very aggressive and appropriate treatment with a combination of laser, injections, and surgery. Definitive treatment with PPV, necessary membrane peeling and simultaneous endo-laser with gas or silicone oil treatment may ameliorate this condition and provide good long-term good vision.

On the bright side, "People with proliferative retinopathy have less than a 5% chance of becoming blind within 5 years when they get timely and appropriate treatment. Although treatments have high success rates, they do not cure diabetic retinopathy" (http://www.nei.nih.gov/health/diabetic/retinopathy.asp).

References

1. National Center for Health Statistics. Health, United States, 2008.
2. Special Eurobarometer, Health in the European Union, September 2007.
3. Gunn RM. Ophthalmoscopic evidence of (1) arterial changes associated with chronic renal diseases and (2) of increased arterial tension. Trans Ophthalmol Soc UK. 1892;12:124–5.
4. Keith NM, Wagener HP, Barker NW. Some different types of essential hypertension: their course and prognosis. Am J Med Sci. 1974;268(6):336–45.
5. Walsh JB. Hypertensive retinopathy. Description, classification, and prognosis. Ophthalmology. 1982;89(10):1127–31.
6. Sharp PS, Chaturvedi N, Wormald R, McKeigue PM, Marmot MG, McHardy Young S. Hypertensive retinopathy in Afro-Caribbeans and Europeans. Prevalence and risk factor relationships. Hypertension. 1995;25:1322–5.
7. Tso MO, Jampol LM. Pathophysiology of hypertensive retinopathy. Ophthalmology. 1982;89(10):1132–45.
8. Hayreh SS, Servais GE, Virdi PS. Fundus lesions in malignant hypertension V. Hypertensive optic neuropathy. Ophthalmology. 1986;93(1):74–87.
9. Lewis RA, Norton EW, Gass JD. Acquired arterial macroaneurysms of the retina. Br J Ophthalmol. 1976;60(1):21–30.
10. Panton RW, Goldberg MF, Farber M. Retinal arterial macroaneurysms: risk factors and natural history. Br J Ophthalmol. 1990;74(10):595–600.
11. Kishi S, Tso MO, Hayreh SS. Fundus lesions in malignant hypertension. I. A pathologic study of experimental hypertensive choroidopathy. Arch Ophthalmol. 1985;103(8):1189–97.
12. Marcucci R, Sofi F, Grifoni E, Sodi A, Prisco D. Retinal vein occlusions: a review for the internist. Intern Emerg Med. 2011;6(4):307–14.
13. Hayreh SS, Podhajsky PA, Zimmerman MB. Retinal artery occlusion associated systemic and ophthalmic abnormalities. Ophthalmology. 2009;116(10):1928–36.
14. Baker ML, Hand PJ, Wang JJ, Wong TY. Retinal signs and stroke: revisiting the link between the eye and brain. Stroke. 2008;39(4):1371–9.
15. Baker ML, Hand PJ, Liew G, Wong TY, Rochtchina E, Mitchell P, Lindley RI, Hankey GJ, Wang JJ, Multi-Centre Retinal Stroke Study Group Stroke. Retinal microvascular signs may provide clues to the underlying vasculopathy in patients with deep intracerebral hemorrhage. Stroke. 2010;41(4):618–23.
16. Lindley RI, Wang JJ, Wong MC, Mitchell P, Liew G, Hand P, Wardlaw J, De Silva DA, Baker M, Rochtchina E, Chen C, Hankey GJ, Chang HM, Fung VS, Gomes L, Wong TY, Multi-Centre Retina and Stroke Study (MCRS) Collaborative Group. Retinal microvasculature in acute lacunar stroke: a cross-sectional study. Lancet Neurol. 2009;8(7):628–34.
17. De Silva DA, Manzano JJ, Liu EY, Woon FP, Wong WX, Chang HM, Chen C, Lindley RI, Wang JJ, Mitchell P, Wong TY, Wong MC, On behalf of the Multi-Centre Retinal Stroke Study Group Neurology. Retinal microvascular changes and subsequent vascular events after ischemic stroke. Neurology. 2011;77(9):896–903.
18. Henderson AD, Bruce BB, Biousse V, Newman NJ. Hypertension-related eye abnormalities and the risk of stroke. Rev Neurol Dis. 2011;8(1–2):1–9.
19. Hayreh SS, Joos KM, Podhajsky PA, et al. Systemic diseases associated with nonarteritic anterior ischemic optic neuropathy. Am J Ophthalmol. 1994;118:766–80.
20. Jacsobson DM, Vierkant RA, Belongia EA. Nonarteritic anterior ischemic optic neuropathy. A case-control study of potential risk factors. Arch Ophthalmol. 1997;115:1403–7.
21. National Society to Prevent Blindness. Vision problems in the US: a statistical analysis. New York: National Society to Prevent Blindness, 1980.
22. Diabetes Control and Complications Trial Research Group. The effect of intensive treatment of diabetes on the development and progression of long-term complications in insulin-dependent diabetes mellitus. N Engl J Med. 1993;329:936–77.

23. Engerman R, Bloodworth JJ. Experimental diabetic retinopathy in dogs. Arch Ophthalmol. 1965;73:205–10.
24. Diabetic Retinopathy Vitrectomy Study Research Group. Early vitrectomy for severe vitreous hemorrhage in diabetic retinopathy: ten year results of a randomized clinical trial, diabetic retinopathy vitrectomy study report no. 2. Arch Ophthalmol. 1985;103:1644–52.
25. Early Treatment of Diabetic Retinopathy Study Research Group. Photocoagulation for diabetic macular edema: ETDRS study report number 1. Arch Ophthalmol. 1985;103:1796–806.
26. Early Treatment of Diabetic Retinopathy Study Research Group. Early photocoagulation for diabetic retinopathy. Ophthalmology. 1991;98:766–85.
27. Aiello LP, Avery RL, Arrigg PG, et al. Vascular endothelial growth factor in ocular fluid of patients with diabetic retinopathy and other retinal disorders. N Engl J Med. 1994;331:1480–7.
28. Kim I, Ryan A, Rohan R, Amano S, Agular S, Miller J, Adamis A. Constiutive expression of VEGF, VEGFR-1, and VEGFR-2 in normal eyes. Invest Ophthalmol Vis Sci. 1999;40(9):2115–21.
29. Diabetic Retinopathy Clinical Research Network (DRCR.net, NIH Roadmap for Medical Research.).
30. Diabetic Retinopathy Study Research Group. Preliminary report on effects of photocoagulation therapy. Am J Ophthalmol. 1976;81:383–96.
31. Diabetic Retinopathy Study Research Group. Photocoagulation treatment of proliferative diabetic retinopathy: the second report of the diabetic retinopathy study findings. Ophthalmology. 1978;85:82–106.

Chapter 9
Predictors of Kidney Disease in Diabetic, Hypertensive Patients

Jaya P. Buddineni, Kunal Chaudhary, and Adam Whaley-Connell

Introduction

Chronic kidney disease (CKD) has global healthcare implications that contribute substantially to an increase in morbidity and mortality. Incident CKD has increased from 12.7% based on data from the National Health and Nutrition Examination Survey (NHANES) III (1988–1994) to 15.1% in 2009 as reported in United States Renal Data System (USRDS) annual report based on NHANES (2003–2006) data. Diabetes is the most common cause of kidney failure in developed and developing nations [1, 2]. Approximate estimates of the global prevalence of diabetes mellitus in 2000 were 2.8% and are expected to grow to 4.4% by 2030, translating to a projected increase of diabetic population from 171 million in 2000 to over 350 million in 2030 [3]. However, hypertension is the most prevalent risk factor for the development of cardiovascular disease (CVD) and augments risk for kidney disease, affecting almost 70 million Americans [1, 4]. In this context, it is widely thought that the presence of hypertension and diabetes augments the risk of individuals for CVD in the general population; this is increasingly recognized to hold true for the development of CKD as well [5].

J.P. Buddineni, M.D.
Department of General Internal Medicine, University of Missouri-Columbia School of Medicine, One Hospital Drive, DC043.00, Columbia, MO 65212, USA
e-mail: buddinenij@health.missouri.edu

K. Chaudhary, M.D. • A. Whaley-Connell, D.O., M.S.P.H. (✉)
Division of Nephrology and Hypertension, Harry S. Truman VA Medical Center, Columbia, MO 65211, USA

Department of Internal Medicine, University of Missouri-Columbia School of Medicine, Columbia, MO 65211, USA
e-mail: chaudharyk@health.missouri.edu; whaleyconnella@health.missouri.edu

S.I. McFarlane and G.L. Bakris (eds.), *Diabetes and Hypertension: Evaluation and Management*, Contemporary Diabetes, DOI 10.1007/978-1-60327-357-2_9,
© Springer Science+Business Media New York 2012

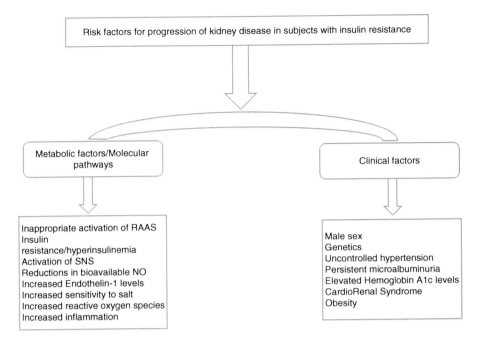

RAAS=Renin Angiotensin Aldosterone System; SNS, Sympathetic nervous System; NO= Nitric Oxide

Fig. 9.1 Metabolic risk factors for kidney disease. *RAAS* renin–angiotensin–aldosterone system, *SNS* sympathetic nervous system, *NO* nitric oxide

There is sufficient evidence to support a strong relationship between hypertension and diabetes pointing towards common genetic and environmental factors that promote their coexistence. Of note, hypertension is noted in almost 50% of diabetic patients at the time of initial diagnosis [6]. According to American Diabetes Association (ADA) clinical practice recommendations, as many as eight million diabetics have undiagnosed hypertension [7]. In a large prospective cohort study of 12,550 subjects, the development of type 2 diabetes mellitus was almost 2.5 times likely in persons noted to have hypertension compared to normotensive subjects [8, 9]. The presence of both hypertension and diabetes mellitus predisposes to the development of CKD and CVD [5, 10] with substantial increase in the risk for coronary heart diseases, stroke, nephropathy, and retinopathy [11, 12]. The underlying mechanisms of each serve to promote the other, thus potentially increasing the risk for development and progression of complications [9, 10]. The association between diabetes and hypertension leads to a biologic common assumption that the underlying mechanisms overlap and involve a common cluster of risk factors.

Increasing evidence suggests that insulin resistance and compensatory hyperinsulinemia may be the link between this complex relationship (Fig. 9.1). Resistance to the metabolic actions of insulin in cardiovascular tissue, namely, heart, vasculature, and even the kidney, contributes to inappropriate activation of RAAS and SNS, inappropriate salt and volume expansion, and increases in tissue inflammation and oxidative stress implicated in the development of proteinuria and CKD [13, 14].

Effect of Hyperinsulinemia on Endothelial Dysfunction

Insulin resistance and compensatory hyperinsulinemia have been related to endothelial dysfunction leading to hypertension [15]. Insulin has a direct impact on endothelial cells and vascular smooth muscle cells (VSMC) via different mechanisms that contribute to endothelial function. Insulin stimulates production of bioavailable nitric oxide (NO) through the phosphatidylinositol 3-kinase (PI3-K)/protein kinase B/Akt pathways in endothelial cells [16]. Further, insulin acts via mitogen-activated protein kinase (MAPK) to stimulate migration and growth of VSMC [17]. Defects in either of these mechanisms due to resistance to the metabolic actions of insulin may result in endothelial dysfunction and manifest as hypertension. Further, NO-dependent vasodilatory mechanisms are impaired in insulin resistance due to imbalance in production and inactivation. Moreover, a free-radical scavenger, super-oxide dismutase (SOD), is suppressed in hypertensive subjects associated with insulin resistance. In addition, an endogenous competitive inhibitor of NO synthase, asymmetric dimethylarginine (ADMA), is elevated in hypertension associated with insulin resistance [18]. The cumulative effects of the above changes result in increased oxidative stress, increased formation of reactive oxygen species (ROS), and endothelial dysfunction, thus contributing to the development of hypertension in insulin resistance subjects [19]. The various alterations that contribute to endothelial dysfunction and VSMC proliferation lead to atherosclerosis and hypertension in insulin resistance parallels the similar changes noted in diabetic-related glomerulosclerosis resulting in proteinuria.

Endothelin-1, another product secreted by glomerular endothelial, mesangial, and tubular epithelial cells, has been associated with diminished glomerular filtration, mesangial cell proliferation, and sodium and water retention [20, 21]. Increasing endothelin-1 concentrations have been reported in patients with insulin resistance or hypertension and proteinuria, suggesting a possible role in the development of diabetic kidney disease [22, 23]. Stimulation of protein kinase C regulated phospholipase D, which hydrolyzes phospholipid molecules leading to the formation of phosphatidic acids that stimulate mesangial cell proliferation, is one of the several mechanisms implicated in endothelin-1 leading [24] to renal injury. However, further research is needed to better understand the complex interplay between insulin and endothelin-1 in kidneys.

The Link Between Insulin Resistance/Hyperinsulinemia, Hypertension, and CKD

Epidemiological studies noted a strong relationship between hypertension and diabetes pointing towards common genetic and environmental factors in promoting both and leading to progression of complications. The clustering of insulin resistance and central obesity contributing to pro-thrombotic and pro-inflammatory abnormalities is well noted [25]. The increase in insulin resistance/hyperinsulinemia contributes to alterations in metabolic signaling pathways that lead to inappropriate activation of the renin–angiotensin–aldosterone system (RAAS) activation and the sympathetic nervous system (SNS) with subsequent increased tissue inflammation and reactive oxygen species (ROS) production leading to endothelial dysfunction that manifests as hypertension.

Alternatively, approximately 25–47% of patients with hypertension have insulin resistance or impaired glucose tolerance [26]. Thereby, the association between hypertension and insulin resistance is very complex and bidirectional. Untreated patients with essential hypertension have been noted to have higher fasting and postprandial insulin levels than normotensive patients regardless of body mass, thus emphasizing the correlation between plasma insulin levels and hypertension [27]. In contrary to the above findings, the relationship between hyperinsulinemia and hypertension has not been noted in some forms of secondary hypertension [27], indicating that insulin resistance is not a consequence of hypertension but supports a common genetic predisposition for both. The above findings are further reinforced by the observation of abnormal glucose metabolism in the offspring of hypertensive individuals [28].

Preclinical data suggest that the diabetic-related kidney injury in early stages occurs during hyperinsulinemia and not overt hyperglycemia and the onset of overt diabetes (Fig. 9.2) [28, 29]. Experimental studies have noted the deleterious effects of persistent elevation of insulin, leading to impairment of renal hemodynamics such as insulin-mediated vasodilation and increased renal plasma flow thus causing rise in glomerular filtration in hypertensive individuals [30, 31]. Elevated insulin levels are also noted to cause sodium retention in vascular system and salt sensitivity thus leading to increased glomerular pressure, hyperfiltration, and urinary albumin excretion (UAE) in diabetic subjects [32]. The normal production of nitric oxide (NO) mediated by insulin through activation of phosphatidylinositol 3-kinase signaling pathways is deranged in an insulin resistant state. The decreasing concentrations of NO and myosin light chain activation add to the derangement of Na^+–K^+ exchange, resulting in increased intracellular calcium concentration, thus potentially to the development of vasoconstriction and intraglomerular hypertension and increased UAE [33]. Few past studies have also noted a strong association between angiotensin II (Ang II), hypertension, and diabetes [34, 35]. Recent evidence from various studies demonstrates that activation of RAS with increased Ang II and oxidative stress are involved in podocyte injury in animal models with hyperinsulinemia [36, 37]. Hyperglycemia, per se, is noted to induce Ang II in podocytes through upregulation of angiotensinogen expression [38]. Consistent with the hyperglycemic state, exposure to in vitro protein along with mechanical stretch to mimic intraglomerular hypertension enhances Ang II production, thus potentiating the impact of hyperinsulinemia on glomerular injury.

Insulin has shown to promote mesangial proliferation, along with synthesis of proteins that regulate extracellular matrix and basement membrane deposition leading to renal injury [39]. Furthermore, insulin via effects of TGF-β on mesangium and proximal tubule cells contribute to the development of microalbuminuria and CKD [40, 41].

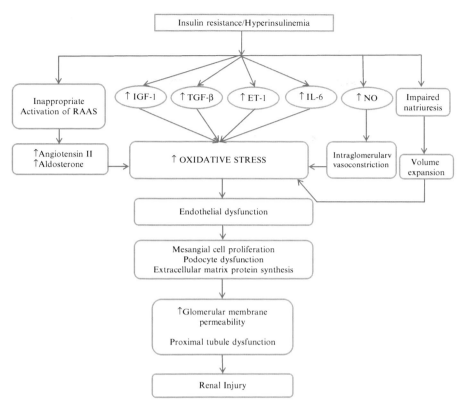

RAAS=Renin Angiotensin Aldosterone System; IGF-1=Insulin like growth factor-1; TGF-β=Transforming growth factor-β; ET-1=Endothelin-1; IL-6=Interluekin-6; NO= Nitric Oxide

Fig. 9.2 Mechanisms relating Insulin resistance and kidney disease. *RAAS* renin–angiotensin–aldosterone system, *IGF-*1 insulin like growth factor-1, *TGF-*β transforming growth factor-β, *ET-*1 endothelin-1, *IL-*6 interluekin-6, *NO* nitric oxide

Effects of Hyperinsulinemia on Sodium and Extracellular Fluid Retention

Various mechanisms have been noted in the ability of renal sodium and extracellular fluid (ECF) handling in patients with insulin resistance that contributes to hypertension and ultimately CKD. Insulin, per se, directly increases proximal tubular sodium reabsorption leading to an anti-natriuretic effect in normal, hypertensive, and insulin-resistant obese subjects [42, 43]. Elevated insulin levels are noted to cause suppression of atrial natriuretic peptide (ANP), thus leading to sodium retention [44, 45]. Moreover, subjects with DM and obesity are noted to be excessively sensitive to dietary salt intake, thus contributing to sodium retention and ECF expansion [46].

Effects of Hyperinsulinemia on the Renin–Angiotensin–Aldosterone System

The strong association between hypertension, insulin resistance, and upregulation of the RAAS is well established [34, 35, 47]. Ang II actions on the Ang type 1 receptor contribute to diminished insulin-dependent PI3K/Akt signaling and subsequent impairments in vasodilatation and glucose transport properties [48, 49]. RAAS-mediated increase in oxidative stress is a significant contributing factor for insulin resistance in cardiovascular tissue. This finding is supported by the rise in reactive oxygen species in heart, vascular, and kidney tissue from transgenic Ren2 rats that overexpress tissue levels of Ang II that exhibit reductions in PI3-K/Akt signaling and impairments in insulin-dependent vasodilatation improved with blockade of the AT_1R [49]. These preclinical findings have been supported through multiple clinical investigations demonstrating that angiotensin-converting enzyme inhibitors (ACE-I) or angiotensin receptor blockers (ARB) [50] improve insulin sensitivity and hypertension [51–53]. The increases in aldosterone secretion in response to changes in ECF volume or alterations in salt intake are primarily mediated by Ang II. Both Ang II and aldosterone exert genomic and non-genomic effects on the systemic, cerebral, and renal vasculature that lead to endothelial dysfunction, insulin resistance, and kidney disease [19]. The role of aldosterone has been substantiated by studies wherein aldosterone antagonists improve cardiac diastolic dysfunction and vascular compliance and decrease proteinuria [12].

Effects of Hyperinsulinemia on Increased Sympathetic Nervous System Activity

RAAS activation and endothelial dysfunction have shown to exert a stimulation effect on the SNS primarily through the influence of Ang II on the release of norepinephrine from the sympathetic nerve terminals [54]. Moreover, in obese individuals increased visceral adipose tissue (VAT) predisposes to hyperinsulinemic state through several mechanisms including activation of SNS, anti-natriuretic peptides, and insulin-related peptides [55, 56]. Plasma leptin levels from adipose tissue may also play a significant role in mediating hypertension associated with CMS and obesity [57, 58].

Effects of Insulin Resistance/Hyperinsulinemia on Inflammation and Oxidative Stress

Persistent subclinical elevations of inflammatory markers such as interleukin-6 (IL-6), C-reactive protein (CRP), elevated white blood cell counts, and fibrinogen levels are associated with insulin resistance and ultimately the development of overt diabetes in the adult population, especially in obese subjects [59]. VAT is a significant source of adipocytokines such as Ang II, endothelin, IL-6, IL-1β, tumor necrosis factor-α (TNF-α), renin, and nonesterified fatty acids (NEFA) [60, 61]. It has been proposed that a few of these inflammatory markers act via c-Jun NH2-terminal kinase (JNK)/AP-1 signaling pathways and modulate the expression of genes coding for inflammatory proteins, thus altering insulin signaling and leading to decrease in insulin sensitivity [59]. A few of the above adipocytokines have shown to cause HTN via direct pressor actions and interactions with RAAS and SNS [62].

Risk Factors for Prediction of Incident CKD in Insulin Resistance and Hypertension

It is thought that persistent microalbuminuria (defined as urinary albumin excretion rate between 30 and 300 mg per 24 h) is a risk factor for development of overt diabetic kidney disease [63]. In a prospective, observational study done in type 1 diabetic subjects, baseline factors associated with progression to persistent microalbuminuria were urinary albumin excretion rate, male, elevations in mean arterial blood pressure, and hemoglobin A1c concentration [64]. Urinary albumin excretion rate, even within normal range at baseline, has shown to be a strong predictor of progressive renal disease [64, 65]. Thus, patients with decreased renal functional reserve are more prone to persistent MAU when exposed to conditions such as hypertension or hyperglycemia. It has also been noted that short stature leading to impaired intrauterine growth results in fewer nephrons, ultimately leading to glomerular hypertension in adulthood [66]. Further large-scale studies are needed to establish a relationship among the above-mentioned risk factors.

In a follow-up sixth Framingham offspring study examination done in 2,345 participants from 1995 to 1998, a multi-marker approach to predict incident CKD and MA concluded the significant role of circulating homocysteine, aldosterone, and B-type natriuretic peptide (BNP) in predicting risk, beyond the traditional risk factors [67].

Genome-wide association studies (GWAS) have undergone extensive evolution in the past decade for identification of susceptibility foci in kidney disease population. As reported in a recent study, common variants in the region of UMOD gene, which encodes Tamm–Horsfall protein (uromodulin), are associated with CKD. Increasing concentrations of uromodulin have shown to precede the onset of CKD and are associated with a common polymorphism in UMOD region [68]. Furthermore, the identification of two new loci at UBE2E2 on chromosome 3 and in C2CD4A–C2CD4B on chromosome 15 in a Japanese study was associated with susceptibility of type 2 DM population and these results were also replicated in other East Asian population [69]. Further large-scale GWAS studies would be beneficial in better conceptualizing the genetic risk factors in diabetes population.

Management

The Joint National Committee on the Detection, Evaluation, and Treatment of High Blood Pressure (JNC 7) currently recommends a target blood pressure of <130/80 mmHg in those with diabetes and kidney disease [70]. Both pharmacological and non-pharmacological interventions need to be implemented in subjects in whom hypertension is detected. As advocated by the many organizations such as World Health Organization (WHO), International Society of Hypertension (ISH), National Kidney Foundation (NKF)-K/DOQI, and the JNC, the first objective in any hypertensive, diabetic individual at risk for kidney disease should be to initiate lifestyle changes, such as improved diet, regular physical activity, weight loss, and cessation of smoking. The dietary approach to stop hypertension (DASH) eating plan consisting of low-sodium, high-potassium, low-calorie (800–1,500 kcal per day), and high-fiber diet has shown to effectively lower BP [71]. Moreover, numerous studies have demonstrated the significance of modest weight loss to be an effective hypertension management therapy [72]. Along with dietary measures, increasing physical activity such as walking 30–45 min at least for 3–5 days a week has shown to improve lipid profiles, decrease blood pressure, and insulin resistance [71, 73, 74].

Multiple studies have demonstrated the beneficial effects of using certain class of drugs over others in hypertensive diabetic individuals. Data from several large-scale studies such as Captopril Prevention Project (CAPPP) and Heart Outcomes Prevention Evaluation (HOPE) trial have demonstrated the beneficial role of ACE-I in diabetic individuals by improving cardiovascular outcomes, improving insulin sensitivity, and even prevent the development of diabetes in hypertensive individuals by inhibiting RAAS [51, 53, 75]. Furthermore, ACE-I have also shown to slow the progression of nephropathy in microalbuminuric, normotensive type 2 diabetes compared with other antihypertensives [76, 77]. By virtue of its RAAS blockade, Angiotensin Receptor Blockers (ARB) have similar cardioprotective and renal benefits as ACE-I in diabetic hypertensive subjects, but with a better side-effect profile than ACE-I [53]. Data from The Ongoing Telmisartan Alone and in combination with Ramipril Global Endpoint Trial (ONTARGET), a double-blind multicenter study demonstrated no significant advantage when using ACE-I and ARBs together in high-risk diabetes or vascular patients. Moreover, these patients are more prone to hypotensive episodes, when both ACE-I and ARBs are used compared to using either one of them [78]. Thus with available data, combination therapy with ACE-I and ARBs is not routinely recommended and should be reserved in select patient populations. Beta-blockers, in spite of the adverse side-effect profile on glucose and lipid profiles in diabetic obese subjects, are recommended as second line of agents. In fact, carvedilol with both α- and β- receptor blocking properties has shown to increase insulin sensitivity and induce vasodilation [79]. Hence, beta-blockers are more effective when used as a part of multidrug regimen in diabetic subjects. The Antihypertensive and Lipid-Lowering Treatment to Prevent Heart Attack Trial (ALLHAT) concluded the role of thiazide diuretics to be less expensive and superior to ACE-I or Calcium channel blockers in decreasing the incidence of

CVD in hypertensive subjects [80], thus suggesting to be the first line of therapy for hypertensive diabetics, despite the fact that thiazides adversely affect insulin resistance and cause electrolyte imbalances [75]. Supporting this evidence, thiazides have consistently been shown to improve CVD outcomes even in diabetic subjects [81]. Thus, using a diuretic along with ACE-I or ARBs can be a very effective approach to lower BP in diabetic hypertensive subjects.

Conclusions

CKD is an ongoing epidemic in both developing and developed countries leading to an enormous socioeconomic burden on the already limited health resources. Patients with diabetes and hypertension are at substantial higher risk for the development of CKD and CVD. Even though evolving research over the past decade has provided insights into understanding complex relationship between diabetes, hypertension, and the risk for CKD, the residual risk remains high and necessitates further investigation into new directions to reduce the burden of CKD. Patients with both diabetes and hypertension pose an enormous challenge for clinicians and an individualized approach should be utilized taking into account the quality of life, adverse effects of antihypertensive medications, and other comorbid conditions to aggressively attain the maximal blood pressure reduction and to prevent onset or progression of CKD.

References

1. Nelson RG, Tuttle KR. The new KDOQI clinical practice guidelines and clinical practice recommendations for diabetes and CKD. Blood Purif. 2007;25(1):112–4.
2. Buse JB, Ginsberg HN, Bakris GL, et al. Primary prevention of cardiovascular diseases in people with diabetes mellitus: a scientific statement from the American Heart Association and the American Diabetes Association. Diabetes Care. 2007;30(1):162–72.
3. Wild S, Roglic G, Green A, Sicree R, King H. Global prevalence of diabetes: estimates for the year 2000 and projections for 2030. Diabetes Care. 2004;27(5):1047–53.
4. Stamler J, Stamler R, Neaton JD. Blood pressure, systolic and diastolic, and cardiovascular risks. US population data. Arch Intern Med. 1993;153(5):598–615.
5. El-Atat F, McFarlane SI, Sowers JR. Diabetes, hypertension, and cardiovascular derangements: pathophysiology and management. Curr Hypertens Rep. 2004;6(3):215–23.
6. McFarlane SI, Jacober SJ, Winer N, et al. Control of cardiovascular risk factors in patients with diabetes and hypertension at urban academic medical centers. Diabetes Care. 2002;25(4): 718–23.
7. Arauz-Pacheco C, Parrott MA, Raskin P. Hypertension management in adults with diabetes. Diabetes Care. 2004;27 Suppl 1:S65–7.
8. Gress TW, Nieto FJ, Shahar E, Wofford MR, Brancati FL. Hypertension and antihypertensive therapy as risk factors for type 2 diabetes mellitus. Atherosclerosis risk in communities study. N Engl J Med. 2000;342(13):905–12.
9. National High Blood Pressure Education Program Working Group report on hypertension in diabetes. Hypertension. 1994;23(2):145–158; discussion 159–160.

10. Sowers JR. Treatment of hypertension in patients with diabetes. Arch Intern Med. 2004;164(17):1850–7.
11. Bakris GL, Williams M, Dworkin L, et al. Preserving renal function in adults with hypertension and diabetes: a consensus approach. National Kidney Foundation Hypertension and Diabetes Executive Committees Working Group. Am J Kidney Dis. 2000;36(3):646–61.
12. Sowers JR, Haffner S. Treatment of cardiovascular and renal risk factors in the diabetic hypertensive. Hypertension. 2002;40(6):781–8.
13. Rahmouni K, Correia ML, Haynes WG, Mark AL. Obesity-associated hypertension: new insights into mechanisms. Hypertension. 2005;45(1):9–14.
14. Vaz M, Jennings G, Turner A, Cox H, Lambert G, Esler M. Regional sympathetic nervous activity and oxygen consumption in obese normotensive human subjects. Circulation. 1997;96(10):3423–9.
15. Caballero AE. Endothelial dysfunction in obesity and insulin resistance: a road to diabetes and heart disease. Obes Res. 2003;11(11):1278–89.
16. Kuboki K, Jiang ZY, Takahara N, et al. Regulation of endothelial constitutive nitric oxide synthase gene expression in endothelial cells and in vivo: a specific vascular action of insulin. Circulation. 2000;101(6):676–81.
17. Hsueh WA, Quin MJ. Role of endothelial dysfunction in insulin resistance. Am J Cardiol. 2003;92(4A):10J–7.
18. Williams SB, Cusco JA, Roddy MA, Johnstone MT, Creager MA. Impaired nitric oxide-mediated vasodilation in patients with non-insulin-dependent diabetes mellitus. J Am Coll Cardiol. 1996;27(3):567–74.
19. McFarlane SI, Sowers JR. Cardiovascular endocrinology 1: aldosterone function in diabetes mellitus: effects on cardiovascular and renal disease. J Clin Endocrinol Metab. 2003;88(2):516–23.
20. Kohan DE. Endothelins in the kidney: physiology and pathophysiology. Am J Kidney Dis. 1993;22(4):493–510.
21. Marsen TA, Schramek H, Dunn MJ. Renal actions of endothelin: linking cellular signaling pathways to kidney disease. Kidney Int. 1994;45(2):336–44.
22. Lee YJ, Shin SJ, Tsai JH. Increased urinary endothelin-1-like immunoreactivity excretion in NIDDM patients with albuminuria. Diabetes Care. 1994;17(4):263–6.
23. De Mattia G, Cassone-Faldetta M, Bellini C, et al. Role of plasma and urinary endothelin-1 in early diabetic and hypertensive nephropathy. Am J Hypertens. 1998;11(8 Pt 1):983–8.
24. Simonson MS, Herman WH. Protein kinase C and protein tyrosine kinase activity contribute to mitogenic signaling by endothelin-1. Cross-talk between G protein-coupled receptors and pp 60c-src. J Biol Chem. 1993;268(13):9347–57.
25. Chaudhary K, Buddineni JP, Nistala R, Whaley-Connell A. Resistant hypertension in the high-risk metabolic patient. Curr Diab Rep. 2011;11(1):41–6.
26. Reaven GM. Banting lecture 1988. Role of insulin resistance in human disease. Diabetes. 1988;37(12):1595–607.
27. Sechi LA, Melis A, Tedde R. Insulin hypersecretion: a distinctive feature between essential and secondary hypertension. Metabolism. 1992;41(11):1261–6.
28. Reaven GM. Insulin resistance/compensatory hyperinsulinemia, essential hypertension, and cardiovascular disease. J Clin Endocrinol Metab. 2003;88(6):2399–403.
29. Cusumano AM, Bodkin NL, Hansen BC, et al. Glomerular hypertrophy is associated with hyperinsulinemia and precedes overt diabetes in aging rhesus monkeys. Am J Kidney Dis. 2002;40(5):1075–85.
30. Cohen AJ, McCarthy DM, Stoff JS. Direct hemodynamic effect of insulin in the isolated perfused kidney. Am J Physiol. 1989;257(4 Pt 2):F580–5.
31. Dengel DR, Goldberg AP, Mayuga RS, Kairis GM, Weir MR. Insulin resistance, elevated glomerular filtration fraction, and renal injury. Hypertension. 1996;28(1):127–32.
32. Catalano C, Muscelli E, Quinones Galvan A, et al. Effect of insulin on systemic and renal handling of albumin in nondiabetic and NIDDM subjects. Diabetes. 1997;46(5):868–75.

33. McFarlane SI, Banerji M, Sowers JR. Insulin resistance and cardiovascular disease. J Clin Endocrinol Metab. 2001;86(2):713–8.
34. Richey JM, Ader M, Moore D, Bergman RN. Angiotensin II induces insulin resistance independent of changes in interstitial insulin. Am J Physiol. 1999;277(5 Pt 1):E920–6.
35. Ogihara T, Asano T, Ando K, et al. Angiotensin II-induced insulin resistance is associated with enhanced insulin signaling. Hypertension. 2002;40(6):872–9.
36. Coward RJ, Welsh GI, Yang J, et al. The human glomerular podocyte is a novel target for insulin action. Diabetes. 2005;54(11):3095–102.
37. Shepherd PR, Kahn BB. Glucose transporters and insulin action–implications for insulin resistance and diabetes mellitus. N Engl J Med. 1999;341(4):248–57.
38. Gloy J, Henger A, Fischer KG, et al. Angiotensin II depolarizes podocytes in the intact glomerulus of the rat. J Clin Invest. 1997;99(11):2772–81.
39. Conti FG, Striker LJ, Lesniak MA, MacKay K, Roth J, Striker GE. Studies on binding and mitogenic effect of insulin and insulin-like growth factor I in glomerular mesangial cells. Endocrinology. 1988;122(6):2788–95.
40. Nicholas SB. Advances in pathogenetic mechanisms of diabetic nephropathy. Cell Mol Biol (Noisy-le-Grand). 2003;49(8):1319–25.
41. Anderson PW, Zhang XY, Tian J, et al. Insulin and angiotensin II are additive in stimulating TGF-beta 1 and matrix mRNAs in mesangial cells. Kidney Int. 1996;50(3):745–53.
42. Sowers JR, Sowers PS, Peuler JD. Role of insulin resistance and hyperinsulinemia in development of hypertension and atherosclerosis. J Lab Clin Med. 1994;123(5):647–52.
43. Standley PR, Bakir MH, Sowers JR. Vascular insulin abnormalities, hypertension, and accelerated atherosclerosis. Am J Kidney Dis. 1993;21(6 Suppl 3):39–46.
44. Feldt-Rasmussen B, Mathiesen ER, Deckert T, et al. Central role for sodium in the pathogenesis of blood pressure changes independent of angiotensin, aldosterone and catecholamines in type 1 (insulin-dependent) diabetes mellitus. Diabetologia. 1987;30(8):610–7.
45. Weidmann P, Beretta-Piccoli C, Trost BN. Pressor factors and responsiveness in hypertension accompanying diabetes mellitus. Hypertension. 1985;7(6 Pt 2):II33–42.
46. Sowers JR. Effects of insulin and IGF-I on vascular smooth muscle glucose and cation metabolism. Diabetes. 1996;45 Suppl 3:S47–51.
47. Brenner BM, Cooper ME, de Zeeuw D, et al. Effects of losartan on renal and cardiovascular outcomes in patients with type 2 diabetes and nephropathy. N Engl J Med. 2001;345(12):861–9.
48. Sloniger JA, Saengsirisuwan V, Diehl CJ, et al. Defective insulin signaling in skeletal muscle of the hypertensive TG(mREN2)27 rat. Am J Physiol Endocrinol Metab. 2005;288(6):E1074–81.
49. Blendea MC, Jacobs D, Stump CS, et al. Abrogation of oxidative stress improves insulin sensitivity in the Ren-2 rat model of tissue angiotensin II overexpression. Am J Physiol Endocrinol Metab. 2005;288(2):E353–9.
50. McFarlane SI, Kumar A, Sowers JR. Mechanisms by which angiotensin-converting enzyme inhibitors prevent diabetes and cardiovascular disease. Am J Cardiol. 2003;91(12A):30H–7.
51. Niklason A, Hedner T, Niskanen L, Lanke J. Development of diabetes is retarded by ACE inhibition in hypertensive patients–a subanalysis of the captopril prevention project (CAPPP). J Hypertens. 2004;22(3):645–52.
52. Kjeldsen SE, Westheim AS, Os I. Prevention of cardiovascular events and diabetes with angiotensin-receptor blockers in hypertension: LIFE, SCOPE, and VALUE. Curr Hypertens Rep. 2005;7(3):155–7.
53. Scheen AJ. Renin-angiotensin system inhibition prevents type 2 diabetes mellitus. Part 1. A meta-analysis of randomised clinical trials. Diabetes Metab. 2004;30(6):487–96.
54. Grassi G. Renin-angiotensin-sympathetic crosstalks in hypertension: reappraising the relevance of peripheral interactions. J Hypertens. 2001;19(10):1713–6.
55. Kidambi S, Kotchen JM, Grim CE, et al. Association of adrenal steroids with hypertension and the metabolic syndrome in blacks. Hypertension. 2007;49(3):704–11.

56. Sechi LA, Bartoli E. Molecular mechanisms of insulin resistance in arterial hypertension. Blood Press Suppl. 1996;1:47–54.
57. Hall JE, da Silva AA, do Carmo JM, et al. Obesity-induced hypertension: role of sympathetic nervous system, leptin, and melanocortins. J Biol Chem. 2010;285(23):17271–6.
58. Morgan DA, Thedens DR, Weiss R, Rahmouni K. Mechanisms mediating renal sympathetic activation to leptin in obesity. Am J Physiol Regul Integr Comp Physiol. 2008;295(6): R1730–6.
59. Duncan BB, Schmidt MI, Pankow JS, et al. Low-grade systemic inflammation and the development of type 2 diabetes: the atherosclerosis risk in communities study. Diabetes. 2003;52(7):1799–805.
60. Katagiri H, Yamada T, Oka Y. Adiposity and cardiovascular disorders: disturbance of the regulatory system consisting of humoral and neuronal signals. Circ Res. 2007;101(1):27–39.
61. Tilg H, Moschen AR. Adipocytokines: mediators linking adipose tissue, inflammation and immunity. Nat Rev Immunol. 2006;6(10):772–83.
62. Fernandez-Real JM, Ricart W. Insulin resistance and chronic cardiovascular inflammatory syndrome. Endocr Rev. 2003;24(3):278–301.
63. Parving HH, Oxenboll B, Svendsen PA, Christiansen JS, Andersen AR. Early detection of patients at risk of developing diabetic nephropathy. A longitudinal study of urinary albumin excretion. Acta Endocrinol (Copenh). 1982;100(4):550–5.
64. Hovind P, Tarnow L, Rossing P, et al. Predictors for the development of microalbuminuria and macroalbuminuria in patients with type 1 diabetes: inception cohort study. Br Med J. 2004;328(7448):1105.
65. Hostetter TH, Rennke HG, Brenner BM. The case for intrarenal hypertension in the initiation and progression of diabetic and other glomerulopathies. Am J Med. 1982;72(3):375–80.
66. Brenner BM, Chertow GM. Congenital oligonephropathy and the etiology of adult hypertension and progressive renal injury. Am J Kidney Dis. 1994;23(2):171–5.
67. Fox CS, Gona P, Larson MG, et al. A multi-marker approach to predict incident CKD and microalbuminuria. J Am Soc Nephrol. 2010;21(12):2143–9.
68. Kottgen A, Hwang SJ, Larson MG, et al. Uromodulin levels associate with a common UMOD variant and risk for incident CKD. J Am Soc Nephrol. 2010;21(2):337–44.
69. Yamauchi T, Hara K, Maeda S, et al. A genome-wide association study in the Japanese population identifies susceptibility loci for type 2 diabetes at UBE2E2 and C2CD4A-C2CD4B. Nat Genet. 2010;42(10):864–8.
70. Chobanian AV, Bakris GL, Black HR, et al. Seventh report of the Joint National Committee on Prevention, Detection, Evaluation, and Treatment of High Blood Pressure. Hypertension. 2003;42(6):1206–52.
71. Sacks FM, Svetkey LP, Vollmer WM, et al. Effects on blood pressure of reduced dietary sodium and the Dietary Approaches to Stop Hypertension (DASH) diet. DASH-Sodium Collaborative Research Group. N Engl J Med. 2001;344(1):3–10.
72. Wassertheil-Smoller S, Blaufox MD, Oberman AS, Langford HG, Davis BR, Wylie-Rosett J. The Trial of Antihypertensive Interventions and Management (TAIM) study. Adequate weight loss, alone and combined with drug therapy in the treatment of mild hypertension. Arch Intern Med. 1992;152(1):131–6.
73. Halbert JA, Silagy CA, Finucane P, Withers RT, Hamdorf PA. Exercise training and blood lipids in hyperlipidemic and normolipidemic adults: a meta-analysis of randomized, controlled trials. Eur J Clin Nutr. 1999;53(7):514–22.
74. Whelton SP, Chin A, Xin X, He J. Effect of aerobic exercise on blood pressure: a meta-analysis of randomized, controlled trials. Ann Intern Med. 2002;136(7):493–503.
75. Whaley-Connell A, Sowers JR. Hypertension management in type 2 diabetes mellitus: recommendations of the Joint National Committee VII. Endocrinol Metab Clin North Am. 2005;34(1):63–75.
76. Bakris GL, Smith AC, Richardson DJ, et al. Impact of an ACE inhibitor and calcium antagonist on microalbuminuria and lipid subfractions in type 2 diabetes: a randomised, multi-centre pilot study. J Hum Hypertens. 2002;16(3):185–91.

77. Ravid M, Lang R, Rachmani R, Lishner M. Long-term renoprotective effect of angiotensin-converting enzyme inhibition in non-insulin-dependent diabetes mellitus. A 7-year follow-up study. Arch Intern Med. 1996;156(3):286–9.
78. Yusuf S, Teo KK, Pogue J, et al. Telmisartan, ramipril, or both in patients at high risk for vascular events. N Engl J Med. 2008;358(15):1547–59.
79. Giugliano D, Acampora R, Marfella R, et al. Metabolic and cardiovascular effects of carvedilol and atenolol in non-insulin-dependent diabetes mellitus and hypertension. A randomized, controlled trial. Ann Intern Med. 1997;126(12):955–9.
80. ALLHAT Officers and Coordinators for the ALLHAT Collaborative Research Group. The Antihypertensive and Lipid-Lowering Treatment to Prevent Heart Attack Trial. Major outcomes in high-risk hypertensive patients randomized to angiotensin-converting enzyme inhibitor or calcium channel blocker vs diuretic: The Antihypertensive and Lipid-Lowering Treatment to Prevent Heart Attack Trial (ALLHAT). JAMA. 2002;288(23):2981–97.
81. Curb JD, Pressel SL, Cutler JA, et al. Effect of diuretic-based antihypertensive treatment on cardiovascular disease risk in older diabetic patients with isolated systolic hypertension. Systolic Hypertension in the Elderly Program Cooperative Research Group. J Am Med Assoc. 1996;276(23):1886–92.

Chapter 10
Antihypertensive Therapy and New-Onset Diabetes

Ivana Lazich and George L. Bakris

Introduction

Hypertension and type-2 diabetes are frequent comorbidities and require special attention in medical management for adequate prevention of cardiovascular and renal morbidities [1]. The prevalence of both, worldwide, is on the rise and is estimated to reach 29.5% and 5.4%, respectively, of general population by 2025 [2, 3]. This translates into paramount health concern and significant financial burden. It is, therefore, important to recognize factors that play a role in disease development and maintenance. This could potentially be used for the development of improved prevention strategies.

In individuals with hypertension who do not have diabetes, the incidence of diabetes mellitus is higher than those without hypertension [4]. This is partly secondary to clustering of risk factors that include obesity, smoking, physical inactivity, genetic pool, and age. Additionally, however, abundance of data suggests that the choice of antihypertensive treatment can markedly affect the occurrence of diabetes with respect to medication classes used.

Determinants of New Diabetes Onset in Hypertensive Patients

Long-term follow-up of hypertensive patients offers evidence that impaired fasting plasma glucose (FBS), increased body mass index (BMI), age, and uncontrolled hypertension represent major risk factors for diabetes development. Level of

I. Lazich, M.D. • G.L. Bakris, M.D. (✉)
Department of Medicine, ASH Comprehensive Hypertension Center, University of Chicago
Medical Center, 5841 S. Maryland Avenue, MC1027, Chicago, IL 60637, USA
e-mail: gbakris@gmail.com

S.I. McFarlane and G.L. Bakris (eds.), *Diabetes and Hypertension: Evaluation and Management*, Contemporary Diabetes, DOI 10.1007/978-1-60327-357-2_10,
© Springer Science+Business Media New York 2012

hypertensive control is a significant determinant for the risk of diabetes mellitus incidence. In a group of 712 Italian patients with hypertension, individuals with uncontrolled blood pressures had higher incidence of diabetes morbidity (8%) than the groups with at goal pressures (4%) ($p < 0.0001$) even after adjustments for fasting glucose, BMI, or age [5]. Moreover, retrospective analysis of the Rancho Bernardo Study cohort, observed for 8.3 years, provided evidence that not only hypertensives but also prehypertensives tend to have higher risk of diabetes mellitus development even when adjusted for parameters such as BMI, fasting plasma glucose, and insulin sensitivity when compared to normotensives. The increments of 10 mmHg of systolic blood pressure (SBP) increased the risk for future DM by approximately 13% [6]. Other variables, such are FBS, BMI, or age in the context of hypertension and hypertensive treatment, were initially evaluated in participants of large clinical trials such as LIFE (Losartan Intervention For Endpoint Reduction in Hypertension) and CAPPP (The Captopril prevention project). Both groups implemented multivariate regression models finding significant and independent relationship with diabetes onset in hypertensive individuals for all of the above variables [7, 8]. Of interest is that captopril and losartan have delayed and decreased the incidence of diabetes in these subjects with this being more pronounced if there were more variables present. The large cohort of 14,120 patients in Anglo-Scandinavian Cardiac Outcomes Trial–Blood Pressure Lowering Arm (ASCOT–BPLA) has also lent data in support of the above. This group of hypertensives older than 40 and with more than three cardiovascular risk factors was randomized to atenolol-based group and amlodipine-based group with the first being eligible for diuretic addition and the second for angiotensin-converting enzyme inhibitor (ACEI) addition. During a median follow-up of 5.5 years, 1,366 participants developed new-onset diabetes. Presence of elevated fasting glucose, higher BMI, and elevated blood pressures coincided with more frequent diabetes onset. However, the groups assigned to amlodipine and ACEI-based regimen had significantly reduced risk of DM with the number needed to treat of 30 for 5 years for prevention of one diabetic case [9]. Similar findings were observed in a cohort of patients enrolled in VALUE trial (Valsartan Antihypertensive Long term Use Evaluation trial) where the same variables predicted higher incidence of new-onset diabetes. This trial explored 9,995 nondiabetic participants with hypertension on either valsartan or amlodipine through a median follow-up of 4.5 years. The importance of plasma glucose and BMI remained significant in both treatment groups separately but also across the groups with the exclusion of treatment characteristics [10]. Not all studies, however, yielded the same results. The ARIC study (Atherosclerosis Research in Community study) did not find a significant difference in the onset of diabetes with different classes of medications including thiazide diuretics or β blockers [4].

Nevertheless, even though robust, the above data are still derived from trials primarily designed to evaluate other primary outcomes. In addition, potentially important factors such as family history or level of physical activity were omitted and participants were frequently exposed to additional diabetogenic circumstances. Finally, since the groups compared were on different medication regimens, it cannot be discerned if this was a protective effect of RAAS blockers or unwanted effect of diuretics or β blockers. The most important implication stemming from these trials is that the increased risk for new-onset diabetes mellitus could be related to the type of antihypertensive treatment. Considering that the diagnosis of diabetes mellitus is often lifelong and that carries significant health and financial burden, more extensive research, as detailed below, has provided a better insight.

Pharmacotherapeutic Implications

Therapeutic doses of thiazide diuretics and β blockers without vasodilating ability are known to affect glucose metabolism and impair insulin sensitivity [11]. Conversely, calcium channel blockers have neutral effect and renin angiotensin aldosterone system (RAAS) blockers seem to have beneficial outcome [12, 13]. The question remains if these translate into development of diabetes mellitus and if subsequently the administration of these medications should be tailored accordingly. Taylor et al., prospectively explored data from three large cohorts: the Nurses Health Study (NHS) I and II and the Health Professionals Follow up Study (HPFS) evaluated the frequency of DM onset in a span of 8, 10, and 16 years. In the course of the study, 3,589 cases of new DM were recorded and when corrected for usual risk factors, thiazide diuretics treated participants had relative risk of developing this condition of 1.20 (95% CI 1.08–1.33) for older women, 1.45 (1.17–1.79) for younger women, and 1.36 (1.17–1.58) for men. Similarly, β blocker use was shown to have independently a relative risk of 1.32 (95% CI 1.20–1.46) and 1.20 (1.05–1.38) for older women and men, respectively. The use of calcium channel blockers and RAAS blockers was not associated with the increased incidence of DM [14]. In a recent meta-analysis of 34 medical publications, diuretics and/or β blockers were also found to cause higher incidence of new-onset DM. This was particularly evident in individuals with higher risk profiles, i.e., obesity and hypercholesterolemia. However, the analysis did include trials that did not have diabetes incidence as an endpoint and trials that did not separately consider each medication class [15]. Another meta-analysis of trials that included β blockers as a first-line antihypertensive therapy, evaluated the risk for incidental DM in total of 94,492 patients. The findings were consistent with risk increase of 22% for new-onset DM if compared to the group that was on other nondiuretic antihypertensive therapy. This was more pronounced in patients with higher BMIs and impaired fasting glucose [16].

The most convincing evidence comes from a prospective trial where the primary endpoint was change in 2-h oral glucose tolerance test (OGTT) and secondary endpoint was incident diabetes mellitus in 276 glucose-intolerant hypertensive individuals. The comparison was done between patients treated with RAAS blocker/CCB combination vs. RAAS blocker/thiazide diuretic combination. At the study end, a higher incidence of new-onset DM was found in lisinopril/hydrochlorothiazide group at 26.6% vs. trandolapril/verapamil group at 11.0%. In addition, hemoglobin A1 >7% was 10.3% and 1.6%, respectively. Primary end point was also positive for 2 h OGTT change from baseline between groups for 29.7 ± 8.7 mg/dL ($p < 0.001$). The important message from this trial is that thiazide diuretics in patients with impaired fasting glucose negatively affect new-onset DM occurrence. In addition, combination of thiazide diuretics with RAAS blockers does not offer protective effect, as assumed before [17]. The follow-up STAR-LET trial evaluated the reversal of new-onset DM following the replacement of thiazide basement regimen trandolapril-based regimen in a 6-month follow-up. The 2 h OGTT improved from 8.5 ± 3.0 vs. 7.2 ± 2.3 ($p < 0.001$) suggesting that regimen change can improve the risk [18].

An additional observation from the STAR trial is that RAAS blockers have positive impact on normoglycemia. Angiotensin II is known to decrease insulin sensitivity and enhance hepatic glucose production; thus, it is plausible that inhibition of RAAS would provide benefits in glycemic control [19]. Indeed, meta-analyses of trials including ACEIs or ABRs that evaluated risk of new diabetes occurrence found that both classes prevent diabetes [20]. The observation that RAAS blockade prevents diabetes was formally examined more closely in the individuals with impaired fasting glucose treated with ramipril in DREAM trial. This was a prospective randomized placebo-controlled trial with the primary endpoint being the incidence of new-onset DM or death and secondary endpoint of regression to normoglycemia. Even though diabetes occurrence did not significantly differ, there was an increased likelihood of regression to normoglycemia in participants treated with ramipril with a hazard ratio of 1.16 (95% CI 1.07–1.27, $p < 0.001$) [21].

The totality of the evidence, therefore, appears to favor blood pressure control with RAAS blockers and calcium channel blockers over thiazide diuretics and β blockers in individuals who are obese and have impaired fasting glucose. Avoiding thiazide diuretics and β blockers if blood pressure can be controlled with other agents will help stave off development of diabetes mellitus and possibly reverse impaired fasting glucose to normoglycemia. Despite this benefit, there is much uncertainty about their impact on improved cardiovascular morbidity and mortality.

Impact on Cardiovascular Outcomes

Increase in adverse cardiovascular events has been linked to hyperglycemia even without a diagnosis of diabetes [22]. Once diabetes mellitus has been diagnosed, the risk for cardiovascular morbidity and mortality increased to two- to fourfold when compared to healthy individuals [23, 24]. Minimizing the risk or preventing the new-onset diabetes might therefore translate into reduced mortality risk. Different modalities of antihypertensive regimens have not been found to adversely affect major cardiovascular events when compared between diabetics and nondiabetics. Meta-analysis of 27 trials assessed the importance of antihypertensive regimen in diabetic vs. nondiabetic individuals for the development of cardiovascular morbidity. The results did not favor any of the regimens including RAAS blockers, CCB, diuretics, or β blockers with all of them reducing the events comparably

($p>0.19$) [25]. This, however, seems to be different in people who develop hyperglycemia on antihypertensives known to affect glucose control, as evidenced by some observational data [26]. The population-based study, done by Dunder et al., found that participants, who developed increase in blood glucose in the course of antihypertensive treatment with thiazide diuretics or β blockers, were more likely to develop myocardial infarction [27]. This issue was also addressed in SHEP trial (The Systolic Hypertension in Elderly Program) and a long-term follow-up of 14.3 year with, however, somewhat contradictory conclusions. It was found that patients, who were treated with thiazide diuretic and have developed diabetes mellitus in the course of the treatment, had no significant increase in cardiovascular events (adjusted HR 1.043, 95% CI 0.745–1.459) [28]. This finding might be related to the fact that higher incidence of new-onset diabetes mellitus in patients treated with thiazide diuretics evens out in a longer patient follow-up. In ALLHAT (Antihypertensive and Lipid Lowering Treatment to Prevent Heart Attack Trial), even though the diabetes occurrence was more frequent in patients treated with chlorthalidone at the end of 2 years, this did not hold true after 4 years of follow-up. In fact, the risk for incident diabetes mellitus was similar between patient groups treated with different medication classes (i.e., chlorthalidone, lisinopril, and amlodipine) [29].

The difference in cardiovascular endpoints between observational and experimental data may be secondary to different patient populations as well as study designs and additional unaccounted confounding factors. Even more likely is that the proper hypertensive control eliminates the expected rise in cardiovascular risk resulting from the new-onset DM development. The lack of prospective, well-controlled randomized trials that address the outcomes in individuals with incident diabetes mellitus while on antihypertensive therapy prevents definite conclusions at this point.

Conclusion

Concomitant diagnosis of diabetes mellitus and hypertension carries significant risk for adverse outcomes. Treatment modalities available to delay the development of diabetes are preferred since they are associated with lower morbidity. Clinical data suggest that certain classes of antihypertensives such as β blockers and thiazide diuretics can increase the risk of new-onset diabetes mellitus in people who are obese and the elderly if they have impaired fasting glucose. This, however, should not preclude the clinicians from using the thiazide diuretics since this medication category carries substantial benefits in blood pressure lowering potential and stroke reduction in individuals who are hyperinsulinemic and are volume expanded secondary to fluid and sodium retention. Conversely, β blockers have a limited role in hypertensive management particularly as an initial medication and therefore could be easily avoided in individuals at risk unless there is a specific indication for such agent. Newer β blockers with vasodilating properties such as carvedilol, bisoprolol, or nebivolol might be a better choice secondary to their lack of metabolic involvement.

Finally, RAAS blockers are a well-suited regimen associated with decreased risk for DM development, and in patients who have developed glucose impairment on other agents, they can potentially offer reversal. The level of adequate control of blood pressure is likely to offset negative impact if any of the new-onset glucose intolerance or DM in this patient population and should be pursued aggressively.

References

1. Chobanian AV, Bakris GL, Black HR, et al. The Seventh Report of the Joint National Committee on Prevention, Detection, Evaluation, and Treatment of High Blood Pressure: the JNC 7 report. J Am Med Assoc. 2003;289(19):2560–72.
2. Kearney PM, Whelton M, Reynolds K, Muntner P, Whelton PK, He J. Global burden of hypertension: analysis of worldwide data. Lancet. 2005;365(9455):217–23.
3. King H, Aubert RE, Herman WH. Global burden of diabetes, 1995–2025: prevalence, numerical estimates, and projections. Diabetes Care. 1998;21(9):1414–31.
4. Gress TW, Nieto FJ, Shahar E, Wofford MR, Brancati FL. Hypertension and antihypertensive therapy as risk factors for type 2 diabetes mellitus. Atherosclerosis Risk in Communities Study. N Engl J Med. 2000;342(13):905–12.
5. Izzo R, de Simone G, Chinali M, et al. Insufficient control of blood pressure and incident diabetes. Diabetes Care. 2009;32(5):845–50.
6. Kramer CK, von MD, Barrett-Connor E. Mid-life blood pressure levels and the 8-year incidence of type 2 diabetes mellitus: the Rancho Bernardo Study. J Hum Hypertens. 2010;24(8):519–24.
7. Lindholm LH, Ibsen H, Borch-Johnsen K, et al. Risk of new-onset diabetes in the Losartan Intervention for Endpoint reduction in hypertension study. J Hypertens. 2002;20(9):1879–86.
8. Niklason A, Hedner T, Niskanen L, Lanke J. Development of diabetes is retarded by ACE inhibition in hypertensive patients–a subanalysis of the Captopril Prevention Project (CAPPP). J Hypertens. 2004;22(3):645–52.
9. Gupta AK, Dahlof B, Dobson J, Sever PS, Wedel H, Poulter NR. Determinants of new-onset diabetes among 19,257 hypertensive patients randomized in the Anglo-Scandinavian Cardiac Outcomes Trial–Blood Pressure Lowering Arm and the relative influence of antihypertensive medication. Diabetes Care. 2008;31(5):982–8.
10. Aksnes TA, Kjeldsen SE, Rostrup M, Storset O, Hua TA, Julius S. Predictors of new-onset diabetes mellitus in hypertensive patients: the VALUE trial. J Hum Hypertens. 2008;22(8):520–7.
11. Sarafidis PA, Bakris GL. Antihypertensive therapy and the risk of new-onset diabetes. Diabetes Care. 2006;29(5):1167–9.
12. Sarafidis PA, Bakris GL. Do the metabolic effects of beta blockers make them leading or supporting antihypertensive agents in the treatment of hypertension? J Clin Hypertens (Greenwich). 2006;8(5):351–6.
13. Lithell HO. Effect of antihypertensive drugs on insulin, glucose, and lipid metabolism. Diabetes Care. 1991;14(3):203–9.
14. Taylor EN, Hu FB, Curhan GC. Antihypertensive medications and the risk of incident type 2 diabetes. Diabetes Care. 2006;29(5):1065–70.
15. Grimm C, Koberlein J, Wiosna W, Kresimon J, Kiencke P, Rychlik R. New-onset diabetes and antihypertensive treatment. GMS Health Technol Assess. 2010;6:Doc03.
16. Bangalore S, Parkar S, Grossman E, Messerli FH. A meta-analysis of 94,492 patients with hypertension treated with beta blockers to determine the risk of new-onset diabetes mellitus. Am J Cardiol. 2007;100(8):1254–62.

17. Bakris G, Molitch M, Hewkin A, et al. Differences in glucose tolerance between fixed-dose antihypertensive drug combinations in people with metabolic syndrome. Diabetes Care. 2006;29(12):2592–7.
18. Bakris G, Molitch M, Zhou Q, et al. Reversal of diuretic-associated impaired glucose tolerance and new-onset diabetes: results of the STAR-LET study. J Cardiometab Syndr. 2008;3(1):18–25.
19. Scheen AJ. Prevention of type 2 diabetes mellitus through inhibition of the renin-angiotensin system. Drugs. 2004;64(22):2537–65.
20. Gillespie EL, White CM, Kardas M, Lindberg M, Coleman CI. The impact of ACE inhibitors or angiotensin II type 1 receptor blockers on the development of new-onset type 2 diabetes. Diabetes Care. 2005;28(9):2261–6.
21. Bosch J, Yusuf S, Gerstein HC, et al. Effect of ramipril on the incidence of diabetes. N Engl J Med. 2006;355(15):1551–62.
22. Khaw KT, Wareham N, Bingham S, Luben R, Welch A, Day N. Association of hemoglobin A1c with cardiovascular disease and mortality in adults: the European prospective investigation into cancer in Norfolk. Ann Intern Med. 2004;141(6):413–20.
23. Khaw KT, Wareham N, Luben R, et al. Glycated haemoglobin, diabetes, and mortality in men in Norfolk cohort of European prospective investigation of cancer and nutrition (EPIC-Norfolk). Br Med J. 2001;322(7277):15–8.
24. Haffner SM, Lehto S, Ronnemaa T, Pyorala K, Laakso M. Mortality from coronary heart disease in subjects with type 2 diabetes and in nondiabetic subjects with and without prior myocardial infarction. N Engl J Med. 1998;339(4):229–34.
25. Turnbull F, Neal B, Algert C, et al. Effects of different blood pressure-lowering regimens on major cardiovascular events in individuals with and without diabetes mellitus: results of prospectively designed overviews of randomized trials. Arch Intern Med. 2005;165(12):1410–9.
26. Verdecchia P, Reboldi G, Angeli F, et al. Adverse prognostic significance of new diabetes in treated hypertensive subjects. Hypertension. 2004;43(5):963–9.
27. Dunder K, Lind L, Zethelius B, Berglund L, Lithell H. Increase in blood glucose concentration during antihypertensive treatment as a predictor of myocardial infarction: population based cohort study. Br Med J. 2003;326(7391):681.
28. Kostis JB, Wilson AC, Freudenberger RS, Cosgrove NM, Pressel SL, Davis BR. Long-term effect of diuretic-based therapy on fatal outcomes in subjects with isolated systolic hypertension with and without diabetes. Am J Cardiol. 2005;95(1):29–35.
29. Barzilay JI, Davis BR, Cutler JA, et al. Fasting glucose levels and incident diabetes mellitus in older nondiabetic adults randomized to receive 3 different classes of antihypertensive treatment: a report from the Antihypertensive and Lipid-Lowering Treatment to Prevent Heart Attack Trial (ALLHAT). Arch Intern Med. 2006;166(20):2191–201.

Chapter 11
Global Cardiovascular Risk Reduction in People with Diabetes Mellitus and Hypertension

Haisam Ismail and Amgad N. Makaryus

Introduction

Hypertension (HTN) and Diabetes Mellitus (DM) are two of the most prevalent risk factors for Coronary Artery Disease (CAD). Many studies have shown that if Blood Pressure (BP) is well controlled as per The Seventh Report of the Joint National Committee on Prevention, Detection, Evaluation, and Treatment of High Blood Pressure (JNC-7) guidelines to approximately <140/80 mmHg in non-diabetics and to <130/80 mmHg in diabetic hypertensive persons, the risk of cardiovascular disease is lower. However, this hypothesis of intensive BP control is still not supported by solid evidence at this time and we wait to see changes in JNC-8. The main focus of therapy in persons with HTN continues to be to prevent or reduce the incidence of myocardial infarction, congestive heart failure, end stage renal disease, stroke, and death [1–5]. Furthermore, HTN has been demonstrated to be related to insulin resistance and hyperglycemia [6–13]. This has further supported the need to effectively control blood pressure in order to reduce the development of DM and CAD. Similarly, the main focus of therapy in persons with DM is to effectively control blood glucose and to prevent or reduce the incidence of end organ damage. Therapies including angiotensin-converting enzyme inhibitors (ACEi) and statins in the diabetic population have proven to be indispensable by many studies in effecting cardiovascular risk reduction. Several randomized trials have revealed the benefits of calcium channel blockers (CCBs), especially the long acting dihydropyridines. The therapeutic options available to reduce cardiovascular disease risk in patients with DM and HTN will be detailed.

H. Ismail, M.D. • A.N. Makaryus, M.D. (✉)
Department of Cardiology, Hofstra North Shore-LIJ School of Medicine,
North Shore University Hospital, 300 Community Drive, Manhasset, NY 11030, USA
e-mail: amakaryu@nshs.edu

S.I. McFarlane and G.L. Bakris (eds.), *Diabetes and Hypertension: Evaluation and Management*, Contemporary Diabetes, DOI 10.1007/978-1-60327-357-2_11,
© Springer Science+Business Media New York 2012

Hypertension and Its Relation to Cardiovascular Disease

HTN is a major well-known risk factor for CAD in approximately one in four Americans or about 65 million Americans [14, 15]. It has been shown in several studies that it is imperative to effectively control BP in order to reduce the risk of atherosclerotic cardiovascular disease. HTN has been shown to cause endothelial injury leading to a cascade of events mediating the development of atherosclerosis [16]. There are numerous studies that prove lower blood pressure reduces the risk of MI, heart failure, and stroke [6, 7]. There are many classes of antihypertensive medications that help control BP in patients with HTN and several trials compare the different classes.

One of the main mechanisms in the pathogenesis of atherosclerosis and CAD is endothelial injury and decreased vascular compliance caused by HTN [16]. Endothelial injury leads to inflammation and thrombosis by reactive O_2 species and other inflammatory markers [16]. The renin–angiotensin–aldosterone system (RAAS) serves as another mechanism in the etiology of HTN causing CAD as shown in Fig. 11.1. Studies have shown that angiotensin II increases BP and increases the generation of reactive oxygen species which oppose the beneficial effects of nitric oxide and subsequently promote pro-inflammatory factors that contribute to coagulopathy and vascular inflammation [11–13].

Diabetes and Its Relation to Cardiovascular Disease

DM and its micro- and macrovascular complications is a rapidly growing health epidemic [17]. Global data has shown that the prevalence of DM worldwide will reach 439 million by the year 2030 [17]. There are many factors contributing to this epidemic including the aging population, increased survival rates, and the increasing prevalence of obesity. About 40% of newly diagnosed persons with DM have concomitant hypertension, therefore increasing the rate of mortality, stroke, CAD, and precipitating the development of diabetic nephropathy, retinopathy, and neuropathy [18]. Furthermore, several studies have shown that obesity and being overweight increases the risk for CAD in people with DM [19]. Although there has been an increase in the understanding of the pathophysiology of DM, studies have shown that optimal care such as controlling BP, serum lipid levels, and cardiovascular risk management have not been achieved. Obesity is a core issue in the management of DM and therefore promoting weight loss will always be an essential aspect of therapy.

The pathophysiology of DM2 which comprises about 90–95% of persons with DM includes insulin resistance in the liver and skeletal muscles and β-cell dysfunction in the pancreas as shown in Fig. 11.2 [20]. The β cells initially compensate early in the disease by increasing insulin secretion until they are no longer capable, thereby giving rise to increased plasma glucose levels [21]. The Insulin Resistance Atherosclerosis Study (IRAS) study showed that continuous decrease in β-cell

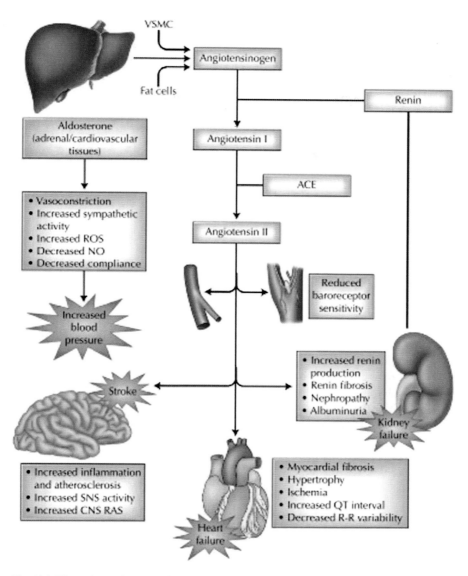

Fig. 11.1 The renin–angiotensin–aldosterone system (RAAS) portraying the effects of angiotensin 2 in the pathogenesis of hypertension. *ACE* angiotensin-converting enzyme, *CNS* central nervous system, *NO* nitric oxide, *ROS* reactive oxygen species, *SNS* sympathetic nervous system, *VSMC* vascular smooth muscle cell. (*From* McFarlane [7]; with permission)

function leads to disease progression [22]. Furthermore, increased glucagon secretion by α-cells in the pancreas contributes to glycemic dysregulation [23]. Recent studies have shown defects in the incretin system as an important pathophysiologic change contributing to the development of DM.

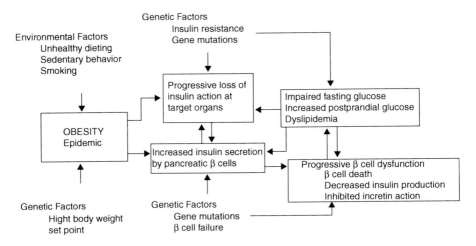

Fig. 11.2 The pathogenesis of diabetes mellitus illustrating the vicious cycle of pancreatic β cell dysfunction and resultant insulin dysregulation. "© 2008 American Diabetes Association From Medical Management of Type 2 Diabetes, Sixth Edition. Reprinted with permission from The American Diabetes Association. To order this book, please call 1-800-232-6455 or order online at http://shopdiabetes.org." [75]

Although DM is associated with an increased risk of CAD, the relative effects of DM on CAD risk in older individuals is less well established [24–29]. The influence of age on the impact of DM on CAD risk is still controversial as older studies suggested a lower mortality risk as age of onset increases [30, 31]. Recent studies have shown that both early and late onset DM are associated with an increased risk for adverse cardiovascular events and that early onset DM for more than 10 years duration as a CAD risk equivalent. This further supports that intensive lifestyle changes and therapy is never too late to prevent adverse cardiovascular events.

Therapeutic Options and Implications

Exercise and Lifestyle Changes

Lifestyle interventions are imperative and should always be an initial part of therapy for persons with HTN and DM [14]. The encouragement of physical activity, healthy dieting, and the cessation of smoking have been shown to prevent the development of CAD [32]. Physical activity and exercise have been proven to enhance the hemodynamic mechanisms in coronary artery flow reserve which is crucial in persons with CAD [33]. Increased afterload due to HTN can extremely impair ventricular relaxation and compromise coronary blood flow during diastole leading to diminished coronary flow reserve [33]. Furthermore, the Look AHEAD (Action for Health in Diabetes) trial investigated an intensive lifestyle intervention in overweight or obese persons with DM. The results of this study inevitably showed significantly improved DM control and CAD risk.

Sedentary behavior is emerging as a new health risk. Recent studies have revealed the detrimental associations of overall sedentary time with dyslipidemia, insulin resistance, and central adiposity leading to an increased risk for the metabolic syndrome [34–38]. The detrimental mechanism proposed by prolonged periods of sitting or sedentary behavior includes fewer skeletal muscle contractions that result in a decreased clearance of triglycerides leading to dyslipidemia, reduced oral glucose load, and less insulin secretion [39–41]. The increase in obesity has resulted in a rising prevalence of DM and therefore, a health awareness of the importance of physical activity that has physicians advising their patients like never before.

Therapy for HTN

Lifestyle modifications may not suffice in persons with HTN and DM. The number and types of antihypertensive agents is over 125 [42]. Many trials have compared the different classes and their combinations in optimal BP management. It is extremely important to adequately control these diseases in order to limit the inevitable progression of cardiovascular disease and ultimately prevent end organ damage.

β-Blockers and Calcium Channel Blockers

β-blockers have been present for many decades and their benefits are well known. Their use has gained some resistance in persons with DM mainly because of metabolic side effects, depression, weight gain, and impotence. The large trial, Glycemic Effects in Diabetes Mellitus: Carvedilol–Metoprolol Comparison in Hypertensives (GEMINI) compared persons already treated with ACEi or angiotensin receptor blockers (ARBs) and either a traditional β-blocker metoprolol or a newer β-blocker carvedilol. The study revealed after approximately 5 months that those treated in the carvedilol arm had a significant reduction in their total cholesterol, triglyceride, and non-high-density lipoprotein cholesterol levels, whereas the metoprolol arm resulted in increased HbA1c by 0.15% and a greater rate of dyslipidemia requiring statin therapy [43]. However, many trials have continued to show that all β blockers not only improve oxygen supply and demand, but also have special anti-arrhythmic properties, cardiac remodeling benefits, and most importantly mortality benefits [44].

Calcium channel blockers (CCBs) have also been around for several decades and more recently have received more support in therapy for persons with HTN. Many trials including ASCOT and INVEST have shown that CCBs specifically the dihydropyridines, are not only comparable to β-blockers but actually even superior in reducing adverse cardiovascular events [45]. In the Trandolapril–Verapamil in Non-insulin Dependent Diabetics (TRAVEND) trial, the ACEi/CCB combination allowed better metabolic control when compared to the ACEi/diuretic combination [46, 47]. CCBs have still been used with caution in persons with HTN, LV dysfunction, and heart failure.

ACE Inhibitors

ACEi and ARBs have been shown to be imperative antihypertensive drugs in treating hypertensive persons with DM. There are many properties beyond BP control in these agents that have been shown in many trials. The Captopril Prevention Project (CAPPP) proved that ACEi lower the risk of MI, stroke, and cardiovascular deaths [10, 45]. Support for the new renin inhibitor aliskiren in the Aliskiren Observation of Heart Failure Treatment (ALOFT) trial showed that not only was BP reduced, but the inherent course of left ventricular disease, heart failure, and proteinuric kidney disease was reduced [48, 49]. Therefore, ACEi, ARBs, and even the newest renin inhibitor aliskiren prove to be essential agents in persons with hypertension and concomitant DM, CAD, and heart failure.

Diuretics

Diuretics especially the thiazides have been used for many years as the initial drugs of choice in controlling BP and reducing cardiovascular risk. The Antihypertensive and Lipid-Lowering Treatment to Prevent Heart Attack Trial (ALLHAT) supported the thiazide diuretics as the first antihypertensive agents of choice. Metabolic side effects have limited their use especially in the elderly. Thiazides have also had diabetogenic effects in some trials which limited their use however, in the large randomized trial Action in Diabetes and Vascular Disease: Preterax and Diamicron MR Controlled Evaluation (ADVANCE), glycemic control did not deteriorate in those treated with ACEi or ARBs and diuretics [50, 51]. Further studies have shown that there was no difference in all cause mortality between the different classes of antihypertensive agents as long as the targeted BP is achieved and end-organ damage is prevented [52]. An algorithm suggesting the treatment combinations in patients with hypertension is illustrated in Fig. 11.3.

Therapy in DM

There are currently five classes of oral DM medications that can be used with or without insulin to adequately control blood sugar. Each agent of a different class targets specific pathophysiologic defects. Therefore, combination therapy can provide optimal results because of complementary mechanisms of action [53].

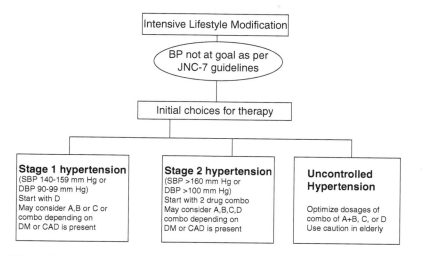

Fig. 11.3 An algorithm suggesting the course of treatment of hypertension with the different classes of therapy. *A* ACEi or ARB, *B* β-blocker, *C* CCB, *D* diuretic. (Adapted from reference [14, 15])

The sulfonylureas are essentially insulin secretagogues. They lower blood glucose levels by stimulating insulin secretion from pancreatic B cells. However, a common side effect of these medications is hypoglycemia [53].

The class of medications known as the thiazolidinediones work by sensitizing the liver and peripheral tissues to insulin therefore attenuating insulin resistance [21, 53]. Side effects really causing a major decline in their use especially seen with rosiglitazone, includes volume retention, heart failure, and MI.

Metformin is a commonly used initial medication for newly diagnosed diabetics. It is a biguanide that suppresses hepatic glucose production in the presence of insulin. Metformin is not associated with hypoglycemia and should not be used in persons with renal failure because of the incidence of lactic acidosis.

The newer medications known as the incretin mimetics work by stimulating the GLP-1 receptors thereby increasing production of insulin in response to high blood glucose levels [54]. A favorable side effect of these agents is weight loss. These are considered by the ADA as tier-2 therapeutic agents. Another class of medications resulting from a better understanding of incretin hormones are the DPP-4 inhibitors. These agents inhibit the degradation of endogenous incretins which increase insulin secretion and decrease glucagon secretion. These medications can cause hypoglycemia and are considered third line agents by the ADA.

Finally, insulin is the most effective hypoglycemic agent and is considered by the ADA as a second agent added after metformin in hard to control diabetics [55].

The main goal of therapy in persons with diabetes is to effectively lower HbA1C levels, not cause hypoglycemia, and to prevent end organ damage.

Therapy in Older Individuals with HTN and DM

There is controversy on the goals of treatment for elderly persons with HTN and DM. Studies have reiterated caution in lowering systolic BP to 130 mmHg in elderly persons with HTN, DM, and CAD because of increased morbidity and mortality. Studies have also continued to discuss the appropriate glycemic target in older patients with DM, because the goals of therapy differ than in younger patients. The goals of therapy for HTN and DM are to reduce morbidity and mortality by decreasing the catastrophic vascular complications such as CAD, stroke, and renal disease. Considering the frailty and overall life expectancy in the elderly, it is imperative to consider the goals of care to each individual patient. For example, moderate control of HTN and DM may provide important benefits such as improved cognition, decreased episodes of hypoglycemia, decreased incontinence, and most importantly decreased falls [56]. This was exemplified in the Action to Control Cardiovascular Risk in Diabetes (ACCORD) trial, which signified that the strategy of intensive glycemic control did not lead to benefits in health related quality of life (HRQL) [57, 58]. The intensive glycemic control arm of the ACCORD trial was actually terminated early because of higher mortality [59]. Furthermore, an INVEST substudy comparing BP and outcomes in very old hypertensive CAD patients revealed that there was no difference in morbidity and mortality between antihypertensive drug treatment strategies [1]. There is a need for further studies determining shorter term outcomes with quality of life for the elderly to help guide clinicians on a patient centered care model for the growing geriatric population.

Pleiotropic Effects of Statins

Statins are a unique class of drugs that are potent inhibitors of cholesterol biosynthesis in the liver by inhibiting the enzyme HMG- CoA reductase. Their role in the primary and secondary prevention of cardiovascular disease has been dramatic. Studies have shown that their role has been more than just lowering lipid levels. They have been shown to improve the risk factors in people with DM and HTN by improving endothelial function, decreasing oxidative stress and inflammation, stabilizing the process of atherosclerosis, and inhibiting thrombogenesis [60]. Studies such as the Cholesterol and Recurrent Events (CARE) and the Heart Protection Study (HPS) have demonstrated that statins indeed have pleiotropic effects that enhance the primary prevention of CAD [61, 62]. Hypercholesterolemia has been proven to be linked with atherosclerosis, which is the main underlying mechanism in CAD. Endothelial dysfunction, an early manifestation of atherosclerosis, is a key process in HTN and DM and statins appear to be key in limiting and preventing this process [63, 64]. Platelets are also known to play a critical role in acute coronary syndrome and CAD, and although the mechanism is not clearly understood, statins have been shown to influence platelet function and inhibit the thrombogenic response [65, 66]. Statins have been shown to decrease plaque size and modify the lipid core of these plaques, therefore contributing to plaque stability and preventing their inevitable rupture [67, 68]. Increased inflammation by way of inflammatory cytokines is a process that contributes to atherosclerosis and statins have been proven to lower the clinical markers of inflammation as shown in the CARE study with lower high-sensitivity C-reactive protein levels [69, 70]. Therefore, statins have been an imperative part of therapy in people with DM and HTN in lowering the cardiovascular risk profile.

Summary

The increased prevalence of DM and HTN has led to the global health epidemic of CAD. Obesity and sedentary behavior have been proven by many studies to increase the rates of dyslipidemia, atherosclerosis, insulin resistance, and the metabolic syndrome [34–38]. The pathophysiology of HTN has been shown to cause endothelial dysfunction, progression of atherosclerosis, and even insulin resistance [16]. About 40% of persons with new DM have concomitant HTN [18]. Furthermore, prediabetes, which is defined as impaired fasting glucose levels of 100–125 mg/dL or most recently as HbA1C levels of 5.7–6.4%, has been projected by surveys to include about 65 million Americans [71, 72]. Therefore, intensive lifestyle interventions such as weight loss, exercise, and healthy dieting as evidenced in the Diabetes Prevention Program (DPP) continues to be an integral part of therapy to those at risk, but several studies reiterated that these interventions be within reason and to conform to the HRQL in the growing geriatric population [57, 58, 73, 74]. It is paramount to try to control the progression of HTN and DM in high-risk patients before it is too late. There are several different classes of medications to control BP and blood glucose in those patients with established disease that can prevent the progression of atherosclerotic CAD. Numerous trials have compared therapies in persons with HTN and DM, and the main focus of therapy will always be to prevent end organ damage. Statins are an essential part of therapy in those patients with DM and HTN to prevent the development of CAD. A stepwise approach patient-centered model that includes intensive lifestyle modifications to prevent the development of HTN and DM in those patients at high risk, and appropriate therapy including a RAAS inhibitor and statin in those patients with established disease allows for the prevention of the inevitable progression to CAD.

References

1. Denardo SJ, Gong Y, Nichols WW, et al. Blood pressure and outcomes in very old hypertensive coronary artery disease patients: an INVEST substudy. Am J Med. 2010;123:719–26.
2. Rosamond W, Flegal K, Furie K, et al. American Heart Association Statistics Committee and Stroke Statistics Subcommittee Heart disease and stroke statistics—2008 update: a report from the American Heart Association Statistics Committee and Stroke Statistics Subcommittee. Circulation. 2008;117:e25–146.

3. Sniderman AD, Holme I, Aastveit A, et al. Relation of age, the apolipoprotein B/apolipoprotein A-I ratio, and the risk of fatal myocardial infarction and implications for the primary prevention of cardiovascular disease. Am J Cardiol. 2007;100:217–21.
4. National Center for Health Statistics, Centers for Disease Control and Prevention. Compressed mortality file: underlying cause-of-death, 1979 to 2004.
5. Lewington S, Clarke R, Qizilbash N, et al. Prospective Studies Collaboration Age-specific relevance of usual blood pressure to vascular mortality: a meta-analysis of individual data for one million adults in 61 prospective studies. Lancet. 2002;360:1903–13. Erratum in: Lancet. 361, (9362), 1060 (2003).
6. McFarlane SI, Banerji M, Sowers JR. Insulin resistance and cardiovascular disease. J Clin Endocrinol Metab. 2001;86:713–8.
7. McFarlane SI. Role of angiotensin receptor blockers in diabetes: implications of recent clinical trials. Expert Rev Cardiovasc Ther. 2009;7:1363–71.
8. Sowers JR, Bakris GL. Antihypertensive therapy and the risk of type 2 diabetes mellitus. N Engl J Med. 2000;342:969–70.
9. Tuomilehto J, Lindstrom J, Eriksson JG, et al. Prevention of type 2 diabetes mellitus by changes in lifestyle among subjects with impaired glucose tolerance. N Engl J Med. 2001;344:1343–50.
10. Hansson L, Lindholm LH, Niskanen L, et al. Effect of angiotensin- converting-enzyme inhibition compared with conventional therapy on cardiovascular morbidity and mortality in hypertension: the Captopril Prevention Project (CAPPP) randomised trial. Lancet. 1999;353: 611–6.
11. Yusuf S, Sleight P, Pogue J, et al. Effects of an angiotensin- converting-enzyme inhibitor, ramipril, on cardiovascular events in high-risk patients: the Heart Outcomes Prevention Evaluation Study Investigators. N Engl J Med. 2000;342:145–53.
12. Lindholm LH, Ibsen H, Dahlof B, et al. Cardiovascular morbidity and mortality in patients with diabetes in the Losartan Intervention For Endpoint reduction in hypertension study (LIFE): a randomised trial against atenolol. Lancet. 2002;359:1004–10.
13. Kim S, Iwao H. Molecular and cellular mechanisms of angiotensin II-mediated cardiovascular and renal diseases. Pharmacol Rev. 2000;52:11–34.
14. Chobanian AV, Bakris GL, Black HR, et al. The Seventh Report of the Joint National Committee on Prevention, Detection, Evaluation, and Treatment of High Blood Pressure: the JNC 7 report. J Am Med Assoc. 2003;289:2560–72. This is the JNC 7 guidelines and recommendations.
15. Winer N, Weber MA, Sowers JR. The effect of antihypertensive drugs on vascular compliance. Curr Hypertens Rep. 2001;3:297–304.
16. Oparil S, Zaman MA, Calhoun DA. Pathogenesis of hypertension. Ann Intern Med. 2003;139:761–76.
17. International Diabetes Federation Atlas 2009. Diabetes and impaired glucose tolerance: global burden: prevalence and projections, 2010 and 2030. International Diabetes Federation Web site. http://www.diabetesatlas.org/content/diabetes-and-impaired-glucose-tolerance. Accessed March 11, 2011.
18. Mancia G, De Backer G, Dominiczak A, et al. 2007 Guidelines for the Management of Arterial Hypertension: The Task Force for the Management of Arterial Hypertension of the European Society of Hypertension (ESH) and of the European Society of Cardiology (ESC). J Hypertens. 2007;25:1105–87.
19. National Diabetes Information Clearinghouse (NDIC). National Diabetes statistics, 2007. http://diabetes.niddk.nih.gov/dm/pubs/statistics/. Last update: June 2008. Accessed March 11, 2011.
20. Eeg-Olofsson K, Cederholm J, Nilsson PM, et al. Risk of cardiovascular disease and mortality in overweight and obese patients with type 2 diabetes: an observational study in 13,087 patients. Diabetologia. 2009;52(1):65–73.
21. Defronzo RA. Banting lecture. From the triumvirate to the ominous octet: a new paradigm for the treatment of type 2 diabetes mellitus. Diabetes. 2009;58(4):773–95.

22. Festa A, Williams K, D'Agostino Jr R, et al. The natural course of beta-cell function in nondiabetic and diabetic individuals: the Insulin Resistance Atherosclerosis Study. Diabetes. 2006;55(4): 1114–20.
23. Freeman JS. The pathophysiologic role of incretins. J Am Osteopath Assoc. 2007;107 suppl 3:S6–9.
24. Notoa D, Cefalù AB, Barbagalloa CM, et al. Hypertension and diabetes mellitus are associated with cardiovascular events in the elderly without cardiovascular disease. Results of a 15-year follow-up in a Mediterranean population. Nutr Metab Cardiovasc Dis. 2009;19(5): 321–6.
25. Rashidi A, Sehgal AR, Rahman M, et al. The case for chronic kidney disease, diabetes mellitus, and myocardial infarction being equivalent risk factors for cardiovascular mortality in patients older than 65 years. Am J Cardiol. 2008;102(12):1668–73.
26. Booth GL, Kapral MK, Fung K, et al. Relation between age and cardiovascular disease in men and women with diabetes compared with non-diabetic people: a population-based retrospective cohort study. Lancet. 2006;368(9529):29–36.
27. Lotufo PA, Gaziano JM, Chae CU, et al. Diabetes and all-cause and coronary heart disease mortality among US male physicians. Arch Intern Med. 2001;161(2):242–7.
28. Woodward M, Zhang X, Barzi F, et al. Asia Pacific Cohort Studies Collaboration. The effects of diabetes on the risks of major cardiovascular diseases and death in the Asia-Pacific region. Diabetes Care. 2003;26(2):360–6.
29. Emerging Risk Factors Collaboration, Sarwar N, Gao P, Kondapally S, et al. Fasting glucose concentration, diabetes mellitus, and risk of vascular disease: a collaborative meta-analysis of 102 prospective studies. Lancet. 2010;375:2215–22.
30. Gu K, Cowie CC, Harris MI. Mortality in adults with and without diabetes in a national cohort of the U.S. population, 1971–1993. Diabetes Care. 1998;21(7):1138–45.
31. Barnett KN, McMurdo ME, Ogston SA, et al. Mortality in people diagnosed with type 2 diabetes at an older age: a systematic review. Age Ageing. 2006;35(5):463–8.
32. Rozanski A, Blumenthal JA, Kaplan J. Impact of psychological factors on the pathogenesis of cardiovascular disease and implications for therapy. Circulation. 1999;99(16):2192–217.
33. Hambrecht R, Wolf A, Gielen S, et al. Effects of exercise on coronary endothelial function in patients with coronary artery disease. N Engl J Med. 2000;342:454–60.
34. Healy GN, Wijndaele K, Dunstan DW, et al. Objectively measured sedentary time, physical activity, and metabolic risk: the Australian Diabetes, Obesity and Lifestyle Study (AusDiab). Diabetes Care. 2008;31(2):369–71.
35. Dunstan DW, Salmon J, Healy GN, et al. Association of television viewing with fasting and 2-h postchallenge plasma glucose levels in adults without diagnosed diabetes. Diabetes Care. 2007;30(3):516–22.
36. Ford ES, Li C, Zhao G, et al. Sedentary behavior, physical activity, and concentrations of insulin among US adults. Metabolism. 2010;59(9):1268–75.
37. Healy GN, Dunstan DW, Salmon J, et al. Objectively measured light-intensity physical activity is independently associated with 2-h plasma glucose. Diabetes Care. 2007;30(6):1384–9.
38. Thorp AA, Healy GN, Owen N, et al. Deleterious associations of sitting time and television viewing time with cardiometabolic risk biomarkers: Australian Diabetes, Obesity and Lifestyle (AusDiab) study 2004–2005. Diabetes Care. 2010;33(2):327–34.
39. Hamburg NM, McMackin CJ, Huang AL, et al. Physical inactivity rapidly induces insulin resistance and microvascular dysfunction in healthy volunteers. Arterioscler Thromb Vasc Biol. 2007;27(12):2650–6.
40. Hamilton MT, Hamilton DG, Zderic TW. Role of low energy expenditure and sitting in obesity, metabolic syndrome, type 2 diabetes, and cardiovascular disease. Diabetes. 2007;56(11): 2655–67.
41. Bey L, Hamilton MT. Suppression of skeletal muscle lipoprotein lipase activity during physical inactivity: a molecular reason to maintain daily low-intensity activity. J Physiol. 2003;551 (Pt 2):673–82.

42. Black HR, Greenberg BH, Weber MA. The foundation role of beta blockers across the cardiovascular disease spectrum: a year 2009 update. Am J Med. 2010;123(11):S2.
43. Bell DS, Bakris GL, McGill JB. Comparison of carvedilol and metoprolol on serum lipid concentration in diabetic hypertensive patients. Diabetes Obes Metab. 2009;11(3):234–8.
44. Reboldi G, Gentile G, Angeli F, et al. Exploring the optimal combination therapy in hypertensive patients with diabetes mellitus. Expert Rev Cardiovasc Ther. 2009;7(11):1349–61.
45. Poulter NR, Dobson JE, Sever PS, et al. Baseline Heart Rate, Antihypertensive Treatment, and Prevention of Cardiovascular Outcomes in ASCOT (Anglo-Scandinavian Cardiac Outcomes Trial). J Am Coll Cardiol. 2009;54:1154–61.
46. Fernández R, Puig JG, Rodríguez-Pérez JC, et al. Effect of two antihypertensive combinations on metabolic control in type-2 diabetic hypertensive patients with albuminuria: a randomised, double-blind study. J Hum Hypertens. 2001;15(12):849–56.
47. Holzgreve H, Nakov R, Beck K, et al. Antihypertensive therapy with verapamil SR plus trandolapril versus atenolol plus chlorthalidone on glycemic control. Am J Hypertens. 2003;16(5 Pt 1):381–6.
48. Gradman AH, Kad R. Renin inhibition in hypertension. J Am Coll Cardiol. 2008;51:519–28.
49. Ismail H, Mitchell R, McFarlane S, et al. Pleiotropic effects of inhibitors of the RAAS in the diabetic population: above and beyond blood pressure lowering. Curr Diab Rep. 2010;10(1):32–6.
50. Patel A, MacMahon S, Chalmers J, et al. Effects of a fixed combination of perindopril and indapamide on macrovascular and microvascular outcomes in patients with type 2 diabetes mellitus (the ADVANCE trial): a randomised controlled trial. Lancet. 2007;370(9590): 829–40.
51. Kinouchi K, Ichihara A, Sakoda M, et al. Safety and benefits of a tablet combining losartan and hydrochlorothiazide in Japanese diabetic patients with hypertension. Hypertens Res. 2009;32(12):1143–7.
52. Turnbull F, Neal B, Algert C, et al. Effects of different blood pressure-lowering regimens on major cardiovascular events in individuals with and without diabetes mellitus: results of prospectively designed overviews of randomized trials. Arch Intern Med. 2005;165(12):1410–9.
53. Rodbard HW, Jellinger PS, Davidson JA, et al. Statement by an American Association of Clinical Endocrinologists/American College of Endocrinology consensus panel on type 2 diabetes mellitus: an algorithm for glycemic control. Endocr Pract. 2009;15(6):540–59.
54. Drucker DJ. The biology of incretin hormones. Cell Metab. 2006;3(3):153–65.
55. Nathan DM, Buse JB, Davidson MB, et al. Medical management of hyperglycemia in type 2 diabetes: a consensus algorithm for the initiation and adjustment of therapy: a consensus statement of the American Diabetes Association and the European Association for the Study of Diabetes. Diabetes Care. 2009;32(1):193–203.
56. Lee SJ, Eng C. Golas of glycemic control in frail older patients with diabetes. J Am Med Assoc. 2011;305(13):1350–1.
57. Gerstein HC, Miller ME, Byington RP, et al. Action to Control Cardiovascular Risk in Diabetes Study Group. Effects of intensive glucose lowering in type 2 diabetes. N Engl J Med. 2008;358(24):2545–59.
58. Sullivan MD, Anderson RT, Aron D, et al. Health-related quality of life and cost-effectiveness components of the Action to Control Cardiovascular Risk in Diabetes (ACCORD) trial: rationale and design. Am J Cardiol. 2007;99(12A):90i–102.
59. Riddle MC, Ambrosius WT, Brillon DJ, et al. Action to Control Cardiovascular Risk in Diabetes Investigators. Epidemiologic relationships between A1C and all-cause mortality during a median 3.4-year follow-up of glycemic treatment in the ACCORD trial. Diabetes Care. 2010;33(5):983–90.
60. Liao JK, Laufs U. Pleiotropic effects of statins. Annu Rev Pharmacol Toxicol. 2005;45: 89–118.
61. Sacks FM, Pfeffer MA, Moye LA, et al. The effect of pravastatin on coronary events after myocardial infarction in patients with average cholesterol levels. Cholesterol and Recurrent Events Trial investigators. N Engl J Med. 1996;335:1001–9.

62. Heart Protection Study Collaborative Group. MRC/BHF Heart Protection Study of cholesterol lowering with simvastatin in 20,536 high-risk individuals: a randomised placebo-controlled trial. Lancet. 2002;360:7–22.

63. Liao JK, Bettmann MA, Sandor T, et al. Differential impairment of vasodilator responsiveness of peripheral resistance and conduit vessels in humans with atherosclerosis. Circ Res. 1991;68:1027–34.

64. Libby P. Molecular bases of the acute coronary syndromes. Circulation. 1995;91:2844–50.

65. Huhle G, Abletshauser C, Mayer N, et al. Reduction of platelet activity markers in type II hypercholesterolemic patients by a HMG-CoA-reductase inhibitor. Thromb Res. 1999; 95:229–34.

66. Hale LP, Craver KT, Berrier AM, et al. Combination of fosinopril and pravastatin decreases platelet response to thrombin receptor agonist in monkeys. Arterioscler Thromb Vasc Biol. 1998;18:1643–6.

67. Moreno PR, Falk E, Palacios IF, et al. Macrophage infiltration in acute coronary syndromes. Implications for plaque rupture. Circulation. 1994;90:775–8.

68. Shah PK, Falk E, Badimon JJ, et al. Human monocyte-derived macrophages induce collagen breakdown in fibrous caps of atherosclerotic plaques. Potential role of matrix-degrading metalloproteinases and implications for plaque rupture. Circulation. 1995;92:1565–9.

69. Ridker PM, Rifai N, Pfeffer MA, et al. Long-term effects of pravastatin on plasma concentration of C-reactive protein. The Cholesterol and Recurrent Events (CARE) Investigators. Circulation. 1999;100:230–5.

70. Ridker PM, Rifai N, Pfeffer MA, et al. Inflammation, pravastatin, and the risk of coronary events after myocardial infarction in patients with average cholesterol levels. Cholesterol and Recurrent Events (CARE) Investigators. Circulation. 1998;98:839–44.

71. American Diabetes Association. Standards of medical care in diabetes—2010. Diabetes Care. 2010;33:S11–61.

72. 2007 National Diabetes Fact Sheet. http://Cdc.gov/diabetes/pubs/general07.htm. Accessed March 11, 2011.

73. Karam JG, McFarlane SI. Update on the prevention of type 2 diabetes. Curr Diab Rep. 2011;11(1):56–63.

74. Knowler WC, Barrett-Connor E, Fowler SE, et al. Reduction in the incidence of type 2 diabetes with lifestyle intervention or metformin. N Engl J Med. 2002;346(6):393–403.

75. American Diabetes Association. Pathogenesis. In: Burant CF, editor. Medical management of type 2 diabetes. 6th ed. Alexandria, VA: American Diabetes Association; 2008. p. 17–25.

Chapter 12
Prevention of Type 2 Diabetes: Evidence from Clinical Trials

Jocelyne G. Karam and Samy I. McFarlane

Introduction

Over the past decades, diabetes mellitus has become a major public health challenge given its striking worldwide increase in prevalence and its multiple associated complications and health cost. The International Diabetes Federation estimates that 6.6% of the world population (285 million individuals) have diabetes in 2010 and this number is expected to increase to 7.8% (438 million individuals) by 2030 [1]. In the United States, the 2003–2006 National Health and Nutrition Examination Survey (NHANES) analysis projected 23.6 million American adults or around 7% of the population do have diabetes, of which 5.5 million individuals with undiagnosed diabetes [2]. Although the prevalence of diabetes is known to increase with age, with around 23% of American adults aged 60 years or older being diabetics, the individuals with the highest number of new diagnosis of diabetes belong to the 40–59 years old age group [2]. Moreover, the Center of Disease Control and prevention (CDC) recently estimated that, if current trends continue, one in three US American adults could have diabetes in 2050 [3].

J.G. Karam, M.D.
Division of Endocrinology, Maimonides Medical Center, SUNY-Downstate
College of Medicine, 4802 Tenth Avenue, Brooklyn, NY 11219, USA
e-mail: jkaram@maimonidesmed.org

S.I. McFarlane, M.D., M.P.H., M.B.A. (✉)
Division of Endocrinology, Diabetes and Hypertension, Department of Medicine,
SUNY-Downstate and Kings County Hospital, Brooklyn, NY, USA
e-mail: Samy.McFarlane@downstate.edu

S.I. McFarlane and G.L. Bakris (eds.), *Diabetes and Hypertension: Evaluation and Management*, Contemporary Diabetes, DOI 10.1007/978-1-60327-357-2_12,
© Springer Science+Business Media New York 2012

Type 2 diabetes represents over 90% of diabetes around the world and is thought to be strongly associated with obesity and sedentary lifestyle [4]. Furthermore, while type 1 diabetes has historically been the almost exclusive type of diabetes in children and adolescents, the prevalence of type 2 diabetes has alarmingly increased in this age group to reach more than 50% of diabetes in U.S. adolescents of high-risk ethnicities such as African Americans, Indian Americans, and Asian-Pacific Islanders [2].

Long-term complications of uncontrolled diabetes have classically been subdivided in microvascular (retinopathy, nephropathy, neuropathy) and macrovascular (cardiovascular disease, peripheral vascular disease), in addition to acute complications of hyperglycemia such as ketoacidosis and nonketotic hyperosmolar state. Diabetes is considered to be a leading cause of new cases of blindness, kidney failure, and nontraumatic foot amputations in the United States, and a leading cause of kidney failure worldwide [2, 4]. In addition, diabetic patients have decreased life expectancy and increased mortality rates, with cardiovascular disease leading the causes of mortality in these patients [2].

High cost represents another public challenge in the rising epidemic of diabetes as health cost of a diabetic patient is known to be at least more than twice the health cost of a nondiabetic patient. For example, the estimated cost of diabetes was 174 billion dollars in the United States in 2005 [4].

Given the rising prevalence of diabetes and the devastating nature of this disease, curving the diabetes epidemic becomes a public health priority. Unlike type 1 diabetes, type 2 diabetes is a disease that can potentially be prevented because of both the slow onset of its pathologic process as well as the possibility of clinically identifying patients in prediabetic state, opening thus a window for intervention prior to the onset of the disease. Yet the interventions that could prevent diabetes were to be defined and their efficacy to be studied.

Risk Factors for Type 2 DM

The first step in preventing diabetes consists of recognizing individuals at high risk of developing diabetes (Table 12.1). Age over 45 years, family history of diabetes in a parent or a sibling, history of gestational diabetes, history of Polycystic Ovarian Syndrome, and high-risk ethnicity (Native American, African American, Hispanic American, Pacific Islanders) constitute the major nonmodifiable risk factors of type 2 diabetes. On the other hand, modifiable risk factors include impaired fasting glucose (IFG), impaired glucose tolerance (IGT), obesity, sedentary lifestyle, cardiovascular disease, dyslipidemia, and hypertension [5]. Obesity epidemic and sedentary lifestyle are classically linked to the rising prevalence of type 2 diabetes across different ethnic and age groups. Obesity is at the chore of the metabolic syndrome that includes increased waist circumference, high blood pressure, high triglycerides, low HDL cholesterol, and/or abnormal glucose metabolism. Metabolic syndrome is considered a prediabetic state. Furthermore, patients with hypertension alone are 2.5 times more likely to have diabetes than normotensive individuals [6].

Table 12.1 Risk factors for type 2 diabetes

Modifiable risk factors
- Lifestyle (physical inactivity, high-caloric, high-fat intake, cigarette smoking, urbanization)
- Overweight or obesity (BMI $\geq$ 25 kg/m^2)
- Impaired fasting plasma glucose
- Impaired glucose tolerance
- Dyslipidemia (low HDL cholesterol, high triglycerides)
- Hypertension
- Cardiovascular disease
- Polycystic ovarian syndrome
- Antipsychotic therapy

Nonmodifiable risk factors
- Age > 45 years
- Family history of type 2 diabetes (first-degree relative)
- Ethnicity (e.g., Native Americans, Hispanic Americans, African Americans, Asian Americans, and Pacific Islanders)
- Gestational diabetes
- Delivery of baby weighing more than 4 kg

BMI body mass index, *HDL* high-density lipoprotein

Prediabetes

The development of type 2 diabetes is a continuous pathologic process that starts many years before the diagnosis of diabetes. In fact, obesity and sedentary lifestyle, in combination with genetic predisposition, are known initially to cause insulin resistance and subsequent compensatory hyperinsulinism, probably years before development of abnormal glucose levels [7]. With time, the beta-cell function will progressively decline and fail to overcome insulin resistance resulting in IGT followed by IFG and development of type 2 diabetes. Indeed, Butler et al. [8] demonstrated decreased beta-cell volume in autopsies of obese patients with IFG or type 2 diabetes, when compared to obese individuals with normal glucose tolerance. It is estimated that around 40–70% of beta-cell function is already lost by the time diabetes is clinically diagnosed.

The American Diabetes Association and the American Association of Clinical Endocrinologists define prediabetes as fasting glucose levels of 100–125 mg/dL (IFG) and/or glucose levels of 140–199 mg/dL 2 h after an oral load of 75 g of dextrose (IGT) [9, 10]. Hemoglobin A1C level of 5.7–6.4% was recently added as another diagnosis criteria of prediabetic state [9, 10]. Women with history of gestational diabetes or polycystic ovarian syndrome are also known to be at higher risk of developing diabetes.

Prediabetes is highly prevalent worldwide [1]. It is estimated that 7.9% of the world population or 344 million people have IGT [1]. In the United States, a 2003–2007 survey projected that 57 million American adults are prediabetics [11].

Among the patients diagnosed with either IFG or OGT, approximately 25% progress to diabetes over 3–5 years period [12] and most likely the vast majority would become diabetics if observed for longer periods. The highest rates of progression to diabetes are observed in patients with both IFG and IGT, older age, overweight, or other diabetic risk factors.

Beyond the increased risk of progression to diabetes, prediabetic state has been shown to be already associated with microvascular and macrovascular complications even prior to the onset of diabetes. The Decode Study has demonstrated significant increased mortality in 2,766 individuals with IGT after 7 years of follow-up when compared to normoglycemic patients [13]. In Pima Indians, the incidence of retinopathy greatly increases at a fasting plasma glucose >116 mg/dL, a 2-h plasma glucose of 185 mg/dL or an A1C > 6.0% [14].

Similar increase of microvascular and macrovascular complications at A1C lower than the cutoff used to diagnose diabetes was also observed in the United Kingdom Prospective Diabetes Study (UKPDS) where more than half of the participants had already diabetic tissue damage at the time of diagnosis of diabetes [15].

More than ten randomized controlled diabetes prevention trials were published over the last decade, examining the efficacy of various interventions in preventing the progression to diabetes in a prediabetic population (Table 12.2). The interventions assessed can be divided into lifestyle changes, pharmacotherapy, and surgery. The following sections will describe the different trials published to date in diabetes prevention with an outlook of the national guidelines published in the field.

Lifestyle Changes

The observed strong link between the rising epidemic of obesity and the increased prevalence of type 2 diabetes made lifestyle changes aiming weight reduction the first candidate intervention to prevent diabetes. As expected, weight loss, exercise and diet have all been shown, separately or in combination, to be effective in decreasing the incidence of type 2 diabetes in high-risk patients (Table 12.2) [16–21]. This effect was surprisingly and consistently sustained even several years after cessation of the initial intensive lifestyle intervention (Table 12.3) [22–24].

DaQuing diabetes prevention study was published in 1997 and was one of the earliest prospective diabetes prevention randomized controlled trials [16]. The study was conducted in 33 clinics in China, and included 577 subjects with IGT. Participants were randomly assigned to four groups: high vegetables low sugar/low alcohol diet, exercise, diet plus exercise versus standard of care. At 6 years of follow-up, diabetes incidence was significantly reduced by 46% in the exercise group, by 31% in the diet group, and by 42% in the diet plus exercise group when compared to standard care.

In 2006, 14 years after the end of the initial study and 20 years after the initial interventions, the cumulative incidence of diabetes was 80% in the intervention group and 93% in the control group with annual incidence of diabetes of 7% and 11% respectively and 46% lower incidence of diabetes over 20 years period in lifestyle changes group. These long-term results suggest sustained beneficial effects of lifestyle modifications despite the standardization of treatment for all groups over the post-study 14 years follow-up period [22]. Of note, no significant mortality benefit was observed in the long-term follow-up DaQuing study.

Table 12.2 Major diabetes prevention trials showing significant reduction in progression to type 2 diabetes

Trial	Intervention	Population (number)	NNT	TNT (years)
DPP [18]	Intensive lifestyle changes vs. standard	IFG/IGT; n=3,234	7	3
	Metformin vs. standard		14	3
Finnish DPS [17]	Intensive lifestyle changes vs. standard	IGT; n=522	8	4
DaQuing DPS [16]	Diet vs. Exercise vs. Diet+Exercise vs. Standard[a]	IGT; n=577	4/3.75/5.6[a]	6
TRIPOD [30]	Troglitazone vs. placebo	GD; n=266	15	2.5
DREAM [31]	Rosiglitazone vs. placebo	IFG/IGT; n=5,269	7	3
	Ramipril vs. placebo		NS	NS
ACT NOW [32]	Pioglitazone vs. placebo	IGT; n=602	8	2.2
STOP-NIDDM [35]	Acarbose vs. placebo	IFG/IGT; n=1,429	11	3.3
Voglibose ph 3	Voglibose vs. placebo	IGT; n=1,780	21	3±
NAVIGATOR [39]	Nateglinide vs. placebo	IGT and CV risk; n=9,306	NS	NS
	Valsartan vs. placebo		25	5
CANOE [34]	Metformin+rosiglitazone vs. placebo	IGT; n=207	4	3.9
XENDOS [49]	Xenical vs. placebo	All obese; n=3,305	36	4
		Obese+IGT n=694	10	4

NNT number needed to treat, *TNT* time needed to treat, *IFG* impaired fasting glucose *IGT* impaired glucose tolerance, *GD* previous gestational diabetes, *ACE* angiotensin-converting enzyme, *ARBs* angiotensin receptor blockers, *NS* not significant, *CV risk* increased cardiovascular risk

Trials: *DPP* Diabetes Prevention Program, *FDPS* Finnish Diabetes Prevention Study, *TRIPOD* Troglitazone in the Prevention of Diabetes, *DREAM* Diabetes REduction Assessment with ramipril and rosiglitazone Medications, *ACT NOW* ACTos NOW for Prevention of Diabetes, *STOP-NIDDM* Study TO Prevent Non-Insulin Dependent Diabetes, *NAVIGATOR* Nateglinide And Valsartan in Impaired Glucose Tolerance Outcomes Research, *CANOE* CAnadian Normoglycemia Outcomes Evaluation trial, *XENDOS* XENical in the prevention of Diabetes in Obese Subjects

[a]Respectively ±estimated 3 years (1 year of treatment completed)

Table 12.3 Major diabetes prevention long-term follow-up studies

Trial/follow-up trial	Population	Intervention	RRR intervention period (years)	RRR follow-up period (years)	RRR cumulative (years)
DPPOS [24]	IFG/IGT; $n=3,234$	ILC vs. standard	58% (3 years)	NS	34% (10 years)
		Metformin vs. standard	31% (3 years)	NS	18% (10 years)
F/U of Finnish DPS [23]	IGT; $n=522$	ILC vs. standard	56% (4 years)	36% (3 years)	43% (7 years)
F/U of CDQDPS [22]	IGT; $n=577$	Combined ILC vs. standard	51% (6 years)	–	46% (20 years)

RRR relative risk reduction of progression to diabetes, *IFG* impaired fasting glucose, *IGT* impaired glucose tolerance, *ILC* intensive lifestyle changes, *NS* not significant

Trials: *DPPOS* Diabetes Prevention Program Outcomes Study, *F/U of FDPS* Follow-up of Finnish Diabetes Prevention Study, *F/U of CDQPDS* Follow-up of China DaQuing Diabetes Prevention Study

The Finnish Diabetes Prevention Study published in 2001 enrolled 522 middle-aged overweight subjects with IGT [17]. The participants randomized to the intervention group received individualized counseling aiming to reduce weight, total intake of fat and saturated fat and increase uptake of fiber and physical activity. The control group received standard therapy. At 4 years of follow-up, the cumulative incidence of diabetes was 11% in the intervention group and 23% in the control group, with a 58% reduction of progression to diabetes.

A follow-up of the Finnish Prevention Study was published in 2006 [23]. Participants who did not progress to diabetes in the initial 4-year study were further followed-up for a median of 3 years. Interestingly, lifestyle changes were maintained by the intervention group subjects despite the cessation of the individual counseling, likely explaining at least in part a 36% relative reduction in diabetes incidence during the postintervention follow-up period alone (4.6 vs. 7.2%, $p = 0.041$) and a 43% cumulative diabetes incidence reduction over the 7-year follow-up, demonstrating again the sustained efficacy of lifestyle changes.

The Diabetes Prevention Program (DPP) trial was a landmark NIH-sponsored multicenter randomized controlled trial conducted in the United States and published in 2002 [18]. A total of 3,234 subjects with prediabetes, defined as IFG or IGT, were randomly assigned to intensive lifestyle modification program, metformin 850 mg BID or matching placebo. Lifestyle changes included low fat (<25% of caloric intake) 1,200–1,800 cal diet and exercise for 150 min a week with a 7% body weight reduction goal and a very well structured curriculum and support professional group. A significant superiority of lifestyle changes led to the premature discontinuation of the study with, at 3 years, a relative risk reduction of progression to diabetes of 58% in lifestyle changes group and 31% in metformin group when compared to placebo (cumulative incidence of diabetes of 28.9%, 21.7%, and 14.4% in the placebo, metformin and lifestyle intervention groups respectively). Lifestyle changes were significantly more effective than metformin and were consistent in men and women across ages, BMI, and ethnic groups.

The DPPOS (DPP Outcome Study) was a 10-year follow-up of the DPP study published in 2009 where all participants were offered group-implemented lifestyle changes and were followed for additional 5.7 years [24]. Unlike the Finnish follow-up study, diabetes incidence was similar in the three treatment groups in the follow-up period. However, the cumulative incidence of diabetes remained lowest in the original lifestyle group with 34% cumulative risk reduction in the lifestyle group and 18% reduction in the metformin group at 10 years when compared to placebo. Interestingly, unlike most of other weight-reducing agent studies, lifestyle changes and metformin succeeded to maintain weight loss at 10 years follow-up in the DPPOS study.

Exercise

Exercise is thought to improve insulin sensitivity and promote peripheral glucose uptake in normal individuals. Long-term moderate exercise, similar to the exercise recommended in DPP and Finnish Diabetes Prevention Study, results in increased translocation of insulin-responsive glucose transporter (GLUT-4) from intracellular stores to the cell surface, facilitating glucose uptake [19].

A systematic review of ten prospective cohort studies published in 2007 showed that, after adjustment for BMI, moderate-intensity physical activity was significantly associated with reduced diabetes incidence [20].

In the Finnish Prevention Study, participants who achieved at least 4 h exercise per week had significant decreased incidence of diabetes (RRR = 80%), effect that is consistent even in the group who did not lose weight [17].

In the DaQuing study, the highest reduction of diabetes incidence was observed in the exercise group [16].

Weight Loss

Weight reduction in prediabetic individuals, even at small or moderate scales, has been consistently associated with reduced incidence of diabetes.

For example, within the same lifestyle intervention group in the Finnish Diabetes Prevention Study, the participants who were able to achieve more than 5% of initial body weight reduction at 1 year did significantly progress less to diabetes when compared to their peers in the interventional group who had less or no weight loss and to the control group (odds ratios (OR) 0.3 and 0.4 respectively) [17].

What is particularly clinically relevant in the diabetes prevention trials is that only modest weight reduction is associated with diabetes prevention.

In the DPP trial, an average weight loss of only 5.6 kg was associated with a 58% lower incidence of diabetes [18]. Moreover, on further analysis of the DPP trial, and among weight, diet and exercise, diabetes prevention correlated most strongly with weight loss, with an estimated 16% diabetes risk reduction for every single kilogram of weight reduction [21].

In the Finnish Diabetes Prevention Study, participants who were able to achieve >5% of initial body weight reduction at 1 year progressed less to diabetes (relative risk reduction of 74%) when compared to their peers in the interventional group who had less weight loss.

Pharmacologic Interventions

Metformin

Metformin is an antidiabetic agent that works mostly at the liver site by suppressing hepatic glucose production and inhibiting free fatty acids (FFA) production and oxidation, therefore reducing FFA-induced insulin resistance and promoting peripheral glucose uptake [25].

In the DPP trial, although generally less effective than lifestyle changes, metformin was associated with a significant 31% diabetes incidence risk reduction (risk of 22% in metformin group versus 29% in placebo group at 3 years) and significant weight reduction of an average of 2 kg [18]. Further analysis of the DPP results showed that metformin efficacy compared to placebo was greater in subjects with younger age, higher body mass index (BMI), and higher fasting sugar levels [18]. In addition, a DPP substudy of 350 women with history of gestational diabetes and IGT revealed that this group of women had a higher risk of progression to diabetes (71% at 3 years) when compared to women with no history of gestational diabetes despite similar baseline glucose levels, and had similar risk reduction of 50% with both metformin and lifestyle changes [26].

Of note, a washout study conducted on the DPP participants after 1–2 weeks of discontinuing metformin or placebo indicated that the incidence of diabetes was still reduced by 25% in the metformin group after the washout period, suggesting a partially sustained rather than temporary effect of metformin [27]. In the DPPOS follow-up study, metformin (850 mg BID as tolerated) was continued in the group initially assigned to metformin in addition to lifestyle counseling. The progression to diabetes was similar in all groups during the follow-up period of 5.7 years; however the cumulative incidence of diabetes at 10 years was still reduced in the metformin group by 18%, reflecting a sustained initial risk reduction. Furthermore, the weight loss associated with metformin was also sustained at 10 years [24].

This beneficial effect of metformin observed in the DPP trial was supported by the results of a meta-analysis by Slapeter et al. [28] in 2008 that reported relative risk reduction of new onset diabetes of 40% with metformin.

Therefore, metformin is considered a relatively safe and effective alternative for diabetes prevention should lifestyle changes be insufficient.

Thiazolidinediones

Thiazolidinediones (TZDs) are peroxisome proliferator-activated gamma receptor (PPAR-γ) agonists that work by increasing peripheral insulin sensitivity via augmented conversion of preadipocytes to adipocytes, which in turn increase adiponectin that is associated with increased insulin sensitivity [29]. In addition to their antihyperglycemic properties, TZDs might also have an effect on beta-cell preservation that can ideally translate into prevention and delay of diabetes [30].

The first study to demonstrate diabetes prevention with a TZD was the TRIPOD study (Troglitazone in Prevention of Diabetes) where a total of 266 Hispanic women with history of gestational diabetes were randomly assigned to troglitazone or placebo [30]. Troglitazone use was significantly associated with reduction of progression to diabetes at one and a half-year follow-up when compared to placebo (relative risk reduction of 55%), with a decrease of endogenous insulin requirement at 3 months of therapy and sustained benefit after discontinuation of the TZD, suggesting a potential effect on beta-cell preservation.

Moreover, troglitazone was an investigational drug in the DPP trial from 1996 to 1998 at which time it was discontinued because of associated fatal liver failure in a DPP participant. In the DPP trial, troglitazone was associated with a remarkable decreased progression to diabetes by 75% at 1 year. Troglitazone was withdrawn from the US market in 2000 because of its association with severe hepatotoxicity.

The DREAM (Diabetes REduction Assessment with ramipril and rosiglitazone Medications) trial was one of the largest primary diabetes prevention trials with over 5,000 participants with IFG and/or IGT randomized to rosiglitazone, ramipril or placebo in a 2×2 factorial design [31]. Participants receiving rosiglitazone had 60% less progression to diabetes and 71% more regression to normoglycemia when compared to placebo. However, the use of rosiglitazone was associated with an increased risk of new-onset congestive heart failure and a mean weight gain of 2.2 kg that was though reflecting an increase of the subcutaneous gluteal fat depot rather than visceral fat, with decreased waist-to-hip ratio.

Finally, the Actos Now for Prevention of Diabetes (ACT NOW) trial is a randomized and double-blinded study enrolling 602 patients with IGT, assigned to pioglitazone 45 mg daily or placebo [32]. Over a mean follow-up of 2.6 years, pioglitazone was significantly associated with an annual decrease of progression to diabetes of 72% (2.1% compared to 7.6% in placebo group) and increased conversion to normal glucose tolerance, in addition to a favorable effect on fasting and 2 h blood glucose, HbA1C level, diastolic blood pressure, carotid intima thickness, and HDL cholesterol. The incidence of edema and weight gain was significantly higher in the pioglitazone group as expected.

In June 2011, the French and German medication regulatory agencies suspended the sale of pioglitazone because of a potential increased incidence of bladder cancer with the cumulative exposure to more than 28 g of pioglitazone. In the United States, the Food and Drug Administration (FDA) announced that the use of pioglitazone for more than a year may be associated with an increased risk of bladder cancer and is currently undergoing comprehensive data review on this subject [33].

In summary, the use of TZDs has consistently shown a potent beneficial effect in diabetes prevention but was associated with significant adverse effects, particularly new onset of congestive heart failure, and more recently possible increase of incidence of bladder cancer.

Combination of Metformin and Thiazolidinediones

In the CAnadian Normoglycemia Outcomes Evaluation (CANOE) trial, a total of 207 patients with IGT were randomly assigned to receive combination of metformin (500 mg twice daily) and rosiglitazone (2 mg daily) versus placebo for a median of 3.9 years [34]. The combination therapy was associated with a 66% relative risk reduction of progression to diabetes.

Alpha-glucosidase Inhibitors

By decreasing oral carbohydrate intestinal absorption, alpha-glucosidase inhibitors improve postprandial hyperglycemia and eventually reduce glucose toxicity of pancreatic beta cells. In addition, they have been shown to improve insulin sensitivity in individuals with IGT [35]. Therefore, alpha-glucosidase inhibitors have been examined in many diabetes prevention trials and were found to exert a favorable protective effect in prediabetic population [36].

In a major multicenter placebo-controlled randomized trial, the Study to Prevent Non-Insulin Dependent Diabetes Mellitus (STOP-NIDDM), a total of 1,429 subjects with IGT were randomly assigned to receive acarbose 100 mg three times a day or placebo for 3 years [37] [35]. As expected, diabetes incidence was significantly decreased by 25% in the acarbose group (relative risk of 32.4% vs. 41.5% in acarbose and placebo group respectively) with also a significant increased conversion to normal glucose tolerance. Furthermore, the use of acarbose was associated with a significant decrease of 49% of any cardiovascular event, highlighting the cardiovascular protective effect of improving postprandial hyperglycemia with acarbose. The study was limited by an elevated discontinuation rate (31% in the acarbose group and 19% in the placebo group) most likely related to increased gastrointestinal adverse effects of acarbose. In addition, the diabetes prevention effect does not seem to be sustained as during a 3 months washout period where all patients received placebo, incidence of diabetes in the initial intervention group was higher than in the initial placebo group.

In a more recently published Japanese multicenter randomized double-blind trial, a total of 1,780 patients with IGT were randomized to receive Voglibose, another alpha-glucosidase inhibitor, or placebo [38]. The interim analysis at 48 weeks revealed a significant reduction of progression to diabetes in the Voglibose group.

Nateglinides

Nateglinide is a short-acting insulin secretagogue that is used in the treatment of mostly postprandial hyperglycemia in diabetic patients.

The hypothesis of a protective effect of nateglinide in prediabetic population was examined in the NAVIGATOR study (the NAteglinide and Valsartan in Impaired Glucose Tolerance Outcomes Research), the largest prospective multinational, randomized, double-blinded, placebo-controlled diabetes prevention trial. Nateglinide (30–60 mg three times daily) and valsartan (80–160 mg daily) versus placebo were used in a 2×2 factorial design in 9,306 subjects with IGT and increased risk of cardiovascular events [39]. At 5 years, nateglinide did not reduce the cumulative incidence of diabetes or cardiovascular outcomes when compared to placebo whereas risk of hypoglycemia was significantly increased in the intervention group.

ACE Inhibitors and ARBs

Renin–angiotensin system (RAS) blockade was suggested to have a protective effect in diabetes prevention through secondary or post hoc analysis of major hypertension trails such as ramipril in the Heart Outcomes Prevention Evaluation (HOPE) study, captopril (compared to diuretics and beta blockers in The CAptopril Prevention Project (CAPP)), lisinopril (compared to amlodipine and chlorthalidone in The Antihypertensive and Lipid-Lowering Treatment to Prevent Heart Attack Trial (ALLHAT trial)), losartan (compared to atenolol in the Losartan Intervention For Endpoint reduction in hypertension study (LIFE)), and multiple other randomized controlled trials [40–44].

Therefore, two above-mentioned major trials were designed to examine, as a primary outcome, the effect of RAS inhibition in diabetes prevention in population at risk.

The DREAM trial randomized, in a 2 × 2 factorial design, 5,269 relatively healthy participants with IGT and/or IFG to rosiglitazone, ramipril, or placebo [45]. Although the use of ramipril at a dose of 15 mg daily for 3.5 years did not prevent diabetes significantly, it was associated with a 9%, nonsignificant decrease in new onset of diabetes and a 16%, significant increase in regression of IFG and IGT to normoglycemia, as well as a significant decrease in plasma glucose level 2 h after oral load of glucose (135.1 vs. 140.5 mg/dL) with no improvement of fasting blood glucose.

Similarly, in the NAVIGATOR trial that examined the effect of nateglinide and valsartan on the prevention of diabetes in 9,306 subjects with IGT and increased risk of cardiovascular events, valsartan significantly but slightly reduced the incidence of diabetes at 5 years by 14% when compared to placebo (33 vs. 37%, respectively) with no significant reduction in cardiovascular outcomes [46].

Unlike in the DREAM study, the patients enrolled in the NAVIGATOR trial had established cardiovascular disease or cardiovascular risk factors and assumable elevated RAS activation level. This baseline population difference might explain the more significant effect of RAS inhibition in the NAVIGATOR trial.

The use of ACE inhibitors or ARBs should be encouraged in prediabetic patients when indicated for high blood pressure or cardiovascular disease in view of their probable favorable glycemic effect. This effect is thought to be related to different mechanisms: inhibition of the post-receptor insulin signaling abnormalities, increased blood flow to the skeletal muscle facilitating insulin action, and enhanced differentiation of pre-adipocytes into mature adipocytes, increased pancreatic islet blood perfusion leading to appropriate insulin release and possible partial PPAR-γ activity [47] [46–49].

Xenical

Xenical is a gastrointestinal lipase inhibitor used in weight reduction and weight maintenance.

The possible diabetes prevention benefit of xenical was initially suggested by a retrospective analysis of xenical treatment effects on obese patients with IGT [48]. This finding was subsequently confirmed by a multicenter randomized placebo-controlled study, XENical in the prevention of Diabetes in Obese Subjects (XENDOS) study where 3,305 obese subjects, with normal or impaired glucose tolerance, were randomized to either xenical 120 mg three times a day or placebo, in addition to lifestyle changes for all participants [49]. In the group of patients with IGT (694 subjects), xenical treatment was associated with a 45% risk reduction of progression to diabetes at 4 years (18.8% vs. 28.8% in placebo) whereas participants with baseline normal glucose tolerance had no significant change in incidence of diabetes. On the other hand, weight reduction at 4 years was significantly greater in all patients who received xenical (5.8 kg in intervention group vs. 3 kg in control group). The beneficial effect of xenical in diabetes prevention seems to be additive to the benefit of weight loss. As in many weight reduction trials, this study was limited by the high discontinuation rate in both groups (48% in xenical group and 66% in control group) probably related to insufficient clinical response.

Of note, an alert linking xenical with rare cases of severe liver injury was recently issued by the FDA [50].

Statins

Statins are HMG Co-A reductase inhibitors with potent lipid-lowering properties but also multiple protective pleiotropic and cardiovascular effects, including anti-inflammatory, anti-atherosclerotic, blood pressure lowering as well as possible glucose lowering effects [51].

The initial link of statin use to diabetes incidence was derived from a post hoc analysis of the West of Scotland Coronary Prevention Study (WOSCOPS) where 5,974 nondiabetic patients were followed for development of diabetes that occurred in 139 participants [52]. The use of pravastatin 40 mg daily was associated with 30% reduction of diabetes ($p = 0.042$), effect that seemed to be, not only induced by triglyceride lowering effect, but also potentially due to other anti-inflammatory and anti-atherosclerotic properties of the statins.

However, this protective correlation was not replicated in other statin trials. At the other extreme, the Justification for the Use of Statins in Primary Prevention: an intervention Trial Evaluating Rosuvastatin (JUPITER) suggested that patients treated with rosuvastatin have significantly higher incidence of physician-reported type 2 diabetes [53].

In view of the conflicting data surrounding the relation of statins to incident diabetes, Sattar et al. [54] published recently a meta-analysis that included 13 statin trials with 91,140 participants in whom 4,278 developed diabetes at 4 years. The use of statins was found to be associated with a slight but significant 9% increased risk of diabetes, most prominent in older subjects. It is now thought that such a diabetogenic effect can be due to a direct statin-induced beta-cell dysfunction [55].

Fibric Acid Derivatives (Bezafibrate)

Bezafibrate, a nonselective ligand/activator for PPAR alpha, was found to reduce not only triglycerides, but fasting plasma glucose, fructosamine and hemoglobin A1C levels significantly in type 2 diabetic patients with hyperlipidemia [56]. Different mechanisms of glucose lowering have been suggested with bezafibrates: nonselective activation of PPAR gamma, improving insulin sensitivity and enhancing glucose disposal in adipose tissue and skeletal muscles [57]. Furthermore, bezafibrate treatment was also associated with decreased incidence of diabetes in patients with impaired fasting plasma glucose and in obese nondiabetic patients with normal glycemic levels [58, 59].

In a post hoc analysis of the Bezafibrate Infarction Prevention (BIP) Study, 303 patients with IFG received either 400 mg of bezafibrate daily or placebo [59]. Over a mean follow-up of 6.2 years, development of diabetes was less prevalent (54.4% vs. 42.3%, RRR = 22%) and more delayed (mean 10 months) in the Bezafibrate group compared to placebo. Multivariate analysis identified bezafibrate as an independent predictor of decreased risk of new diabetes development, regardless of BMI and lipid profile.

Surgery

Over the past decade, bariatric surgery has become one of the most efficient interventions in inducing and sustaining weight reduction in severely obese patients, with a net associated benefit in diabetes prevention or remission.

The Swedish Obese Subject Study (SOS) is a prospective nonrandomized cohort study that followed 4,047 obese subjects who underwent gastric surgery or were matched obese control for 2 years, and 1,703 participants among them for more than 10 years [60, 61]. The incidence of diabetes at 2 years was reduced by 32-fold in the group of patients undergoing bariatric surgery as compared to weight-stable obese controls (odds ratio = 0.14). This effect was consistent, although less pronounced at 10 years (odds ratio = 0.25).

In a study published by Pories et al. [62], 150 among 152 obese subjects with IGT who underwent gastric bypass achieved and maintained normal glycemic profile at 14 years of follow-up.

Similarly, in a follow-up of 136 obese subjects with IGT, of whom 109 subjects underwent bariatric surgery, one in the surgical group developed diabetes compared to 6 out of 27 in the control group [63].

In a meta-analysis including studies from 22,094 patients who underwent bariatric surgery, 76.8% had complete resolution of their diabetes [64].

The rapid improvement of glycemic profile after bariatric surgery is thought to be due to oral intake restriction as well as acute hormonal changes related to the exclusion of upper gastrointestinal track such as incretins and ghrelin level variations [65].

Conclusion and Recommendations

The diagnosis of type 2 diabetes is usually preceded by a long period of prediabetic state that constitutes a golden opportunity to identify population at risk and prevent diabetes. Lifestyle changes including dietary changes, moderate weight loss, and moderate physical activity have been established as a safe and efficient intervention to prevent diabetes. Their protective effect seems to be sustained for greater than 10 years after the initial intervention. Pharmacologic agents such as metformin, thiazolidinediones, and alphaglucosidase inhibitors have also been associated with diabetes prevention at various degrees. While metformin seems to be a reasonable therapeutic option for prediabetics not responding to lifestyle changes, the use of thiazolidinediones and alphaglucosidase inhibitors in this context is limited by associated side effects and cost.

RAS blockade and fibrates should be considered in the treatment of hypertension or hyperlipidemia associated with prediabetes.

The most recent guidelines of the American Diabetes Association recommend referring prediabetic patients to an ongoing support program targeting 7% of body weight reduction and at least 150 min a week of moderate physical activity for all patients with IFG, IGT, or A1C of 5.7–6.4% [9, 10]. Metformin should be considered in those at highest risk of diabetes especially those with progressive hyperglycemia despite lifestyle changes. Monitoring of progression to diabetes should be performed yearly.

References

1. International Diabetes Federation. IDF Diabetes Atlas. http://www.diabetesatlas.org/.
2. 2007 National Diabetes Fact Sheet. Available at http://www.cdc.gov/nchs/fastats/diabetes.htm.
3. http://www.cdc.gov/media/pressrel/2010/r101022.html. 2010.
4. World Health Organization (WHO). Fact Sheet No 312 November 2009. Available at http://www.who.int/mediacentre/factsheets/fs312/en/.
5. Karam JG, McFarlane SI. Update on the prevention of type 2 diabetes. Curr Diab Rep. 2011;11(1):56–63.
6. http://www.cdc.gov/diabetes/pubs/general07.htm.
7. Kruszynska YT, Olefsky JM. Cellular and molecular mechanisms of non-insulin dependent diabetes mellitus. J Investig Med. 1996;44(8):413–28.
8. Butler AE, Janson J, Bonner-Weir S, Ritzel R, Rizza RA, Butler PC. Beta-cell deficit and increased beta-cell apoptosis in humans with type 2 diabetes. Diabetes. 2003;52(1):102–10.
9. American Diabetes Association. Standards of medical care in diabetes—2011. Diabetes Care. 2011;34 Suppl 1:S11–61.
10. Handelsman Y, Mechanick JI, Blonde L, et al. American Association of Clinical Endocrinologists Medical Guidelines for Clinical Practice for developing a diabetes mellitus comprehensive care plan. Endocr Pract. 2011;17 Suppl 2:1–53.
11. Nathan DM, Davidson MB, DeFronzo RA, et al. Impaired fasting glucose and impaired glucose tolerance: implications for care. Diabetes Care. 2007;30(3):753–9.
12. Mokdad AH, Ford ES, Bowman BA, et al. Prevalence of obesity, diabetes, and obesity-related health risk factors, 2001. J Am Med Assoc. 2003;289(1):76–9.

13. Glucose tolerance and mortality: comparison of WHO and American Diabetes Association diagnostic criteria. The DECODE study group. European Diabetes Epidemiology Group. Diabetes Epidemiology: Collaborative analysis Of Diagnostic criteria in Europe. Lancet. 1999;354(9179):617–21.

14. Gabir MM, Hanson RL, Dabelea D, et al. Plasma glucose and prediction of microvascular disease and mortality: evaluation of 1997 American Diabetes Association and 1999 World Health Organization criteria for diagnosis of diabetes. Diabetes Care. 2000;23(8):1113–8.

15. Stratton IM, Adler AI, Neil HA, et al. Association of glycaemia with macrovascular and microvascular complications of type 2 diabetes (UKPDS 35): prospective observational study. Br Med J. 2000;321(7258):405–12.

16. Pan XR, Li GW, Hu YH, et al. Effects of diet and exercise in preventing NIDDM in people with impaired glucose tolerance. The Da Qing IGT and Diabetes Study. Diabetes Care. 1997;20(4):537–44.

17. Tuomilehto J, Lindstrom J, Eriksson JG, et al. Prevention of type 2 diabetes mellitus by changes in lifestyle among subjects with impaired glucose tolerance. N Engl J Med. 2001;344(18):1343–50.

18. Knowler WC, Barrett-Connor E, Fowler SE, et al. Reduction in the incidence of type 2 diabetes with lifestyle intervention or metformin. N Engl J Med. 2002;346(6):393–403.

19. Devlin JT. Effects of exercise on insulin sensitivity in humans. Diabetes Care. 1992;15(11):1690–3.

20. Jeon CY, Lokken RP, Hu FB, van Dam RM. Physical activity of moderate intensity and risk of type 2 diabetes: a systematic review. Diabetes Care. 2007;30(3):744–52.

21. Hamman RF, Wing RR, Edelstein SL, et al. Effect of weight loss with lifestyle intervention on risk of diabetes. Diabetes Care. 2006;29(9):2102–7.

22. Li G, Zhang P, Wang J, et al. The long-term effect of lifestyle interventions to prevent diabetes in the China Da Qing Diabetes Prevention Study: a 20-year follow-up study. Lancet. 2008;371(9626):1783–9.

23. Lindstrom J, Ilanne-Parikka P, Peltonen M, et al. Sustained reduction in the incidence of type 2 diabetes by lifestyle intervention: follow-up of the Finnish Diabetes Prevention Study. Lancet. 2006;368(9548):1673–9.

24. Knowler WC, Fowler SE, Hamman RF, et al. 10-year follow-up of diabetes incidence and weight loss in the Diabetes Prevention Program Outcomes Study. Lancet. 2009;374(9702):1677–86.

25. Kirpichnikov D, McFarlane SI, Sowers JR. Metformin: an update. Ann Intern Med. 2002;137(1):25–33.

26. Ratner RE, Christophi CA, Metzger BE, et al. Prevention of diabetes in women with a history of gestational diabetes: effects of metformin and lifestyle interventions. J Clin Endocrinol Metab. 2008;93(12):4774–9.

27. Diabetes Prevention Program Research Group. Effects of withdrawal from metformin on the development of diabetes in the diabetes prevention program. Diabetes Care. 2003;26(4):977–80.

28. Salpeter SR, Buckley NS, Kahn JA, Salpeter EE. Meta-analysis: metformin treatment in persons at risk for diabetes mellitus. Am J Med. 2008;121(2):149–57. e142.

29. El_Atat F, Nicasio J, Clarke L, et al. Beneficial cardiovascular effects of thiazolidinediones. Therapy. 2005;2:113–9.

30. Buchanan TA, Xiang AH, Peters RK, et al. Preservation of pancreatic beta-cell function and prevention of type 2 diabetes by pharmacological treatment of insulin resistance in high-risk Hispanic women. Diabetes. 2002;51(9):2796–803.

31. Gerstein HC, Yusuf S, Bosch J, et al. Effect of rosiglitazone on the frequency of diabetes in patients with impaired glucose tolerance or impaired fasting glucose: a randomised controlled trial. Lancet. 2006;368(9541):1096–105.

32. DeFronzo RA, Tripathy D, Schwenke DC, et al. Pioglitazone for diabetes prevention in impaired glucose tolerance. N Engl J Med. 2011;364(12):1104–15.

33. FDA Safety announcement about pioglitazone. http://www.fda.gov/Drugs/DrugSafety/ucm259150.htm. Accessed July 8, 2011.
34. Zinman B, Harris SB, Neuman J, et al. Low-dose combination therapy with rosiglitazone and metformin to prevent type 2 diabetes mellitus (CANOE trial): a double-blind randomised controlled study. Lancet. 2010;376(9735):103–11.
35. Chiasson JL, Josse RG, Leiter LA, et al. The effect of acarbose on insulin sensitivity in subjects with impaired glucose tolerance. Diabetes Care. 1996;19(11):1190–3.
36. Van de Laar FA, Lucassen PL, Akkermans RP, Van de Lisdonk EH, De Grauw WJ. Alpha-glucosidase inhibitors for people with impaired glucose tolerance or impaired fasting blood glucose. *Cochrane Database Syst Rev.* 2006;(4):CD005061.
37. Chiasson JL, Josse RG, Gomis R, Hanefeld M, Karasik A, Laakso M. Acarbose for prevention of type 2 diabetes mellitus: the STOP-NIDDM randomised trial. Lancet. 2002;359(9323):2072–7.
38. Kawamori R, Tajima N, Iwamoto Y, Kashiwagi A, Shimamoto K, Kaku K. Voglibose for prevention of type 2 diabetes mellitus: a randomised, double-blind trial in Japanese individuals with impaired glucose tolerance. Lancet. 2009;373(9675):1607–14.
39. Holman RR, Haffner SM, McMurray JJ, et al. Effect of nateglinide on the incidence of diabetes and cardiovascular events. N Engl J Med. 2010;362(16):1463–76.
40. Yusuf S, Gerstein H, Hoogwerf B, et al. Ramipril and the development of diabetes. J Am Med Assoc. 2001;286(15):1882–5.
41. Hansson L, Lindholm LH, Niskanen L, et al. Effect of angiotensin-converting-enzyme inhibition compared with conventional therapy on cardiovascular morbidity and mortality in hypertension: the Captopril Prevention Project (CAPPP) randomised trial. Lancet. 1999;353(9153):611–6.
42. ALLHAT Officers and Coordinators for the ALLHAT Collaborative Research Group. The Antihypertensive and Lipid-Lowering Treatment to Prevent Heart Attack Trial. Major outcomes in high-risk hypertensive patients randomized to angiotensin-converting enzyme inhibitor or calcium channel blocker vs diuretic: The Antihypertensive and Lipid-Lowering Treatment to Prevent Heart Attack Trial (ALLHAT). J Am Med Assoc. 2002;288(23):2981–97.
43. Lindholm LH, Ibsen H, Dahlof B, et al. Cardiovascular morbidity and mortality in patients with diabetes in the Losartan Intervention For Endpoint reduction in hypertension study (LIFE): a randomised trial against atenolol. Lancet. 2002;359(9311):1004–10.
44. Gillespie EL, White CM, Kardas M, Lindberg M, Coleman CI. The impact of ACE inhibitors or angiotensin II type 1 receptor blockers on the development of new-onset type 2 diabetes. Diabetes Care. 2005;28(9):2261–6.
45. Bosch J, Yusuf S, Gerstein HC, et al. Effect of ramipril on the incidence of diabetes. N Engl J Med. 2006;355(15):1551–62.
46. McMurray JJ, Holman RR, Haffner SM, et al. Effect of valsartan on the incidence of diabetes and cardiovascular events. N Engl J Med. 2010;362(16):1477–90.
47. McFarlane SI, Kumar A, Sowers JR. Mechanisms by which angiotensin-converting enzyme inhibitors prevent diabetes and cardiovascular disease. Am J Cardiol. 2003;91(12A):30H–7.
48. Heymsfield SB, Segal KR, Hauptman J, et al. Effects of weight loss with orlistat on glucose tolerance and progression to type 2 diabetes in obese adults. Arch Intern Med. 2000;160(9):1321–6.
49. Torgerson JS, Hauptman J, Boldrin MN, Sjostrom L. XENical in the prevention of diabetes in obese subjects (XENDOS) study: a randomized study of orlistat as an adjunct to lifestyle changes for the prevention of type 2 diabetes in obese patients. Diabetes Care. 2004;27(1):155–61.
50. FDA Safety Announcement about xenical. http://www.fda.gov/safety/medwatch/safetyinformation/safetyalertsforhumanmedicalproducts/ucm213448.htm. Accessed July 8, 2011.
51. McFarlane SI, Muniyappa R, Francisco R, Sowers JR. Clinical review 145: pleiotropic effects of statins: lipid reduction and beyond. J Clin Endocrinol Metab. 2002;87(4):1451–8.

52. Freeman DJ, Norrie J, Sattar N, et al. Pravastatin and the development of diabetes mellitus: evidence for a protective treatment effect in the West of Scotland Coronary Prevention Study. Circulation. 2001;103(3):357–62.
53. Ridker PM, Danielson E, Fonseca FA, et al. Rosuvastatin to prevent vascular events in men and women with elevated C-reactive protein. N Engl J Med. 2008;359(21):2195–207.
54. Sattar N, Preiss D, Murray HM, et al. Statins and risk of incident diabetes: a collaborative meta-analysis of randomised statin trials. Lancet. 2010;375(9716):735–42.
55. Sampson UK, Linton MF, Fazio S. Are statins diabetogenic? Curr Opin Cardiol. 2011;26(4): 342–7.
56. Rovellini A, Sommariva D, Branchi A, et al. Effects of slow release bezafibrate on the lipid pattern and on blood glucose of type 2 diabetic patients with hyperlipidaemia. Pharmacol Res. 1992;25(3):237–45.
57. Tenenbaum A, Motro M, Fisman EZ. Dual and pan-peroxisome proliferator-activated receptors (PPAR) co-agonism: the bezafibrate lessons. Cardiovasc Diabetol. 2005;4:14.
58. Tenenbaum A, Motro M, Fisman EZ, et al. Effect of bezafibrate on incidence of type 2 diabetes mellitus in obese patients. Eur Heart J. 2005;26(19):2032–8.
59. Tenenbaum A, Motro M, Fisman EZ, et al. Peroxisome proliferator-activated receptor ligand bezafibrate for prevention of type 2 diabetes mellitus in patients with coronary artery disease. Circulation. 2004;109(18):2197–202.
60. Sjostrom L, Lindroos AK, Peltonen M, et al. Lifestyle, diabetes, and cardiovascular risk factors 10 years after bariatric surgery. N Engl J Med. 2004;351(26):2683–93.
61. Sjostrom CD. Surgery as an intervention for obesity. Results from the Swedish obese subjects study. Growth Horm IGF Res. 2003;13(Suppl A):S22–6.
62. Pories WJ, Swanson MS, MacDonald KG, et al. Who would have thought it? An operation proves to be the most effective therapy for adult-onset diabetes mellitus. Ann Surg. 1995;222(3):339–50. discussion 350–332.
63. Long SD, O'Brien K, MacDonald Jr KG, et al. Weight loss in severely obese subjects prevents the progression of impaired glucose tolerance to type II diabetes. A longitudinal interventional study. Diabetes Care. 1994;17(5):372–5.
64. Buchwald H, Avidor Y, Braunwald E, et al. Bariatric surgery: a systematic review and meta-analysis. J Am Med Assoc. 2004;292(14):1724–37.
65. Tejirian T, Jensen C, Dutson E. Bariatric surgery and type 2 diabetes mellitus: surgically induced remission. J Diabetes Sci Technol. 2008;2(4):685–91.

Chapter 13
Dietary and Lifestyle Approaches to Hypertension in the Population with Diabetes

Lorena Drago

Introduction

Current estimates indicate that 26 million people in the United States have diabetes according to new estimates from the Centers for Disease Control and Prevention (CDC). Type 2 diabetes accounts for 90–95% of diabetes cases. Type 2 diabetes mellitus is associated with an increased risk of premature death from cardiovascular disease (CVD), stroke, and end-stage renal disease. Hypertension is a common comorbidity in patients with type 2 diabetes mellitus. In 2005–2008, of adults aged 20 years or older with self-reported diabetes, 67% had blood pressure greater than or equal to 140/90 mmHg or used prescription medications for hypertension. The coexistence of hypertension and diabetes is strongly associated with CVD, stroke, progression of renal disease, and diabetic nephropathy. Blood pressure control reduces the risk of cardiovascular disease (heart disease or stroke) among people with diabetes by 33–50%, and the risk of microvascular complications (eye, kidney, and nerve diseases) by approximately 33%. In general, for every 10 mmHg reduction in systolic blood pressure, the risk for any complication related to diabetes is reduced by 12%. No benefit of reducing systolic blood pressure below 140 mmHg has been demonstrated in randomized clinical trials. Reducing diastolic blood pressure from 90 to 80 mmHg in people with diabetes reduces the risk of major cardiovascular events by 50% [1]. The Joint National Committee on Prevention, Detection, Evaluation, and Treatment of High Blood Pressure (JNC), the National Kidney Foundation, and the American Diabetes Association provide evidence-based recommendations for the treatment of hypertension in patients with type 2 diabetes

L. Drago, M.S., R.D., C.D.N., C.D.E. (✉)
Diabetes Education Program, Lincoln Medical and Mental Health Center,
71-40 112 Street Suite 404 Forest Hills, New York, NY 11375, USA
e-mail: lorenamsrd@aol.com

S.I. McFarlane and G.L. Bakris (eds.), *Diabetes and Hypertension: Evaluation and Management*, Contemporary Diabetes, DOI 10.1007/978-1-60327-357-2_13,
© Springer Science+Business Media New York 2012

Table 13.1 Lifestyle modification to manage hypertension[a,b]

Modification	Recommendation	Approximate systolic blood pressure reduction (range)
Weight reduction	Maintain normal body weight (body mass index 18.5–24.9 kg/m^2)	5–20 mmHg/10 kg weight loss
Adopt a DASH eating plan	Consume a diet rich in fruits, vegetables, and low-fat dairy products with a reduced content of saturated and total fat	8–14 mmHg
Dietary sodium reduction	Reduce dietary sodium intake to no more than 100 mmol per day (2.4 g sodium or 6 g sodium chloride)	2–8 mmHg
Physical activity	Engage in regular aerobic physical activity such as brisk walking (at least 30 min per day, most days of the week)	4–9 mmHg
Moderation of alcohol consumption	Limit consumption to no more than 2 drinks (1 oz or 30 ml ethanol; e.g., 24 oz beer, 10 oz wine, or 3 oz 80-proof whiskey) per day in most men and to no more than 1 drink per day in women and lighter weight persons	2–4 mmHg

Source: The Seventh Report of the Joint National Committee on Prevention, Detection, Evaluation and Treatment of High Blood Pressure: The JNC 7 Report. Bethesda, MD: National Institutes of Heart, Lung, and Blood Institute: 2003. NIH Publication 03–5231
DASH dietary approaches to stop hypertension
[a]For overall cardiovascular risk reduction, stop smoking
[b]The effect of implementing these modifications are dose and time-dependent, and could be greater for some individuals

mellitus. The effectiveness of medical nutrition therapy for type 1 and type 2 diabetes has been well established. Randomized controlled trials and observational studies of medical nutrition therapy have reported decreases in HbA1C an average of ~1–2%. Some studies also reported improved blood pressure and lipid profiles, and weight management [2].

Joint National Committee on Prevention, Detection, Evaluation, and Treatment of High Blood Pressure [3]

High blood pressure treatment guidelines for hypertension with and without compelling indications including heart failure, postmyocardial infarction, high coronary disease risk, diabetes chronic kidney disease, or recurrent stroke prevention include lifestyle modification.

Lifestyle modification is defined as weight reduction, Dietary Approaches to Stop Hypertension (DASH) plan, regular physical activity, and moderate alcohol intake (Table 13.1).

Weight Reduction and Blood Pressure

Hypertension, obesity, and type 2 diabetes frequently coexist contributing to cardiovascular risk factors. In a recent analysis of the Nurse's Health Study, body mass index (BMI) alone was the most powerful predictor of hypertension. Women with a BMI 25 or greater (healthy BMI is 18.5–24.9 kg/m²) had an adjusted population attributable risk of 40% compared with those with a BMI less than 25 [4].

Overall, dietary intervention studies report that weight reduction has antihypertensive effects. A meta-analysis of randomized controlled trials (RCT) on the influence of weight reduction on blood pressure indicated that blood pressure reduction averaged −1.05 mmHg systolic and −0.92 mmHg diastolic per kilogram of weight loss [5].

Weight loss, as an antihypertensive treatment, may be undermined by weight regain over the long term in a dose–response relationship. There might still be a beneficial effect on risk of incident hypertension even after the weight reduction effect has disappeared [6].

To encourage patients to achieve or maintain a healthy weight, health care professionals should:

- Determine the individual's calorie needs. Calorie needs depend on the person's age, gender, height, weight, and level of physical activity. Many individuals are unaware of the number of calories required to achieve a healthy weight or the caloric values of foods and beverages (Table 13.2). To achieve weight loss, it is common to begin with a 500 daily calorie deficit from the individual estimated calorie need.
- Teach patients how to calculate number of calories consumed in a meal with the assistance of calorie and nutrition information tools and instruct them how to read and interpret the nutrition food labels.
- Encourage physical activity as a way to achieve calorie balance. *The 2008 Physical Activity Guidelines for Americans* [8] recommend that adults between 18 and 64 should avoid sedentary behaviors and should engage in at least 150 min a week of moderate-intensity activity. Some adults may require 300 min per week. Adults should also include muscle-strengthening activities.
- Encourage patients to monitor caloric intake by keeping a food diary. A food diary may track portions consumed, underlying reasons for eating, hunger levels, and cravings.
- Refer patient to a Registered Dietitian for individualized medical nutrition therapy and a diabetes educator for diabetes education management. To find a Registered Dietitian, visit http://www.eatright.org, and to find a diabetes educator, visit http://www.diabeteseducator.org.

Table 13.2 Estimated calorie needs per day by age, gender, and physical activity level [7]

Gender	Age (years)	Physical activity level		
		Sedentary	Moderately active	Active
Female	19–30	1,800–2,000	2,000–2,200	2,400
	31–50	1,800	2,000	2,200
	51+	1,600	1,800	2,000–2,200
Male	19–30	2,400–2,600	2,600–2,800	3,000
	31–50	2,200–2,400	2,400–2,600	2,800–3,000
	51+	2,000–2,200	2,200–2,400	2,400–2,800

Sedentary means a lifestyle that includes only the light physical activity associated with typical day-to-day life. Moderately active means a lifestyle that includes physical activity equivalent to walking about 1.5–3 miles per day at 3–4 miles per hour, in addition to the light physical activity associated with typical day-to-day life. Active means a lifestyle that includes physical activity equivalent to walking more than 3 miles per day at 3–4 miles per hour, in addition to the light physical activity associated with typical day-to-day life

Dietary Approaches to Stop Hypertension Eating Plan

The DASH eating plan has been shown to lower high blood pressure in research studies.

The National Heart, Lung, and Blood Institute (NHLBI) sponsored research studies to study the effect of diet on high blood pressure. The DASH eating plan was efficacious in lowering blood pressure in feeding trials [9]. The addition of exercise and weight loss to the DASH eating plan resulted in even larger blood pressure reductions, greater improvements in vascular and autonomic function, and reduced left ventricular mass in a randomized controlled study of overweight or obese persons with above-normal blood pressure [10].

The DASH eating plan:

- Is low in cholesterol, total fat, and saturated fat
- Emphasizes fruits, vegetables, and fat-free or low-fat milk and milk products
- Is rich in whole grains, fish, poultry, beans, seeds, and nuts
- Contains fewer sweets, added sugars and sugary beverages, and red meats than the typical American diet

The Dietary Guidelines for Americans [11] recommend most Americans reduce daily sodium intake to less than 2,300 mg and that African Americans, persons who are 51 or older, and those of any age who have hypertension, diabetes, or chronic kidney disease further reduce intake to 1,500 mg daily. The 1,500 mg recommendation applies to about half of the US population, including children, and the majority of adults.

The DASH eating plan contains 2,300 mg of daily sodium, which is lower in sodium than the typical American diet. Further reducing sodium to no more than 1,500 mg per day further lowers blood pressure.

The DASH eating plan also includes foods rich in potassium, magnesium, and calcium, as well as protein and fiber. A 2,100 calorie diet DASH eating plan contained 4,700 mg of potassium, 1,250 mg of calcium, 500 mg of magnesium, 95 g (18% calories) of protein, and 30 g of dietary fiber.

Potassium and Blood Pressure

Multiple studies have demonstrated that dietary potassium intake has significantly lowered blood pressure in hypertensive and nonhypertensive patients. Potassium also reduces the cerebrovascular accident (CVA) independent of blood pressure reduction. An intake of 4.7 g of potassium predicts an estimated decrease of 8–15% in CVA and 6–11% in myocardial infarction [12].

The Dietary Guidelines for Americans (2010) recommend an intake of potassium equal to or greater than the Adequate Intake (AI). The AI for potassium is set at 4.7 g (120 mmol) per day. In general, potassium should come only from food sources and not supplements. For an extensive list of the potassium content of selected foods, visit http://www.ars.usda.gov/SP2UserFiles/Place/12354500/Data/SR22/nutrlist/sr22w306.pdf (Table 13.3).

Table 13.3 Potassium, K (mg) content of selected foods

Description	Weight (g)	Common measure	Content per measure
Beet greens, cooked, boiled, drained, without salt	144	1 cup	1,309
Raisins, seedless	145	1 cup	1,086
Potato, baked, flesh and skin, without salt	202	1 potato	1,081
Lima beans, large, mature seeds, cooked, boiled, without salt	188	1cup	955
Fish, halibut, Atlantic and Pacific, cooked, dry heat	159	½ fillet	916
Plantains, raw	179	1 medium	893
Spinach, cooked, boiled, drained without salt	180	1 cup	839
Peas, split, mature seeds, cooked, boiled, without salt	196	1 cup	710
Sweet potato, cooked, baked, in skin, without salt	146	1 potato	694
Yogurt, plain, skim milk, 13 g of protein per 8-oz	227	8-oz container	579
Mushrooms, white, cooked, boiled, drained, without salt	156	1 cup	555
Broccoli, cooked, boiled, drained, without salt	156	1 cup	457
Soup, minestrone, canned, reduced sodium, ready-to-serve	241`	1 cup	448
Cucumber, with peel, raw	301	1 large	442
Melons, cantaloupe, raw	160	1 cup	427
Bananas, raw	118	1 banana	422
Corn, sweet, yellow, canned, vacuum packed, regular pack	210	1 cup	391
Carrots, cooked, boiled, drained, without salt	156	1 cup	367
Peaches, raw	170	1 cup	323
Fish, salmon, sockeye, cooked, dry heat	85	3 oz	319

Adapted from the USDA National Nutrition Database for Standard Reference, Release 22 [13]

Magnesium and Blood Pressure

The DASH Eating Plan is also rich in magnesium, exceeding the Recommended Dietary Allowance (RDA). The RDA for magnesium is 320 mg for women over 31 and 420 mg for men over 31. Magnesium intake is believed to have antihypertensive effects although the evidence has yielded conflicting results [14]. Some studies suggest that magnesium intake is associated with lower blood pressure levels [15]. A study on dietary magnesium intake and risk of incident hypertension among women participating in the Women's Health Study reported a significant inverse association between dietary magnesium intake and blood pressure levels [16]. Replacing sodium chloride with Smart Salt, a mineral salt containing 50% sodium, 25% potassium, and 25% magnesium with high blood pressure resulted in a significant reduction in systolic blood pressure [17]. Most of the evidence suggests that patients with hypertension would benefit from magnesium-rich foods, such as whole grains, nuts, legumes, and green leafy vegetables.

DASH Eating Plan Nutrient Recommendations

The DASH eating plan daily serving recommendations are based on individual caloric needs to achieve or maintain a healthy weight (Table 13.4).

Persons with diabetes who adopt the DASH eating plan should be counseled to emphasize the selection of the healthiest and nutrient-dense foods. When possible, patients should limit foods with added solid fats and added sugars. Encourage patients to select foods from the following food groups.

Carbohydrate

Dietary carbohydrate is the major determinant of postprandial glucose levels. Carbohydrate is found in all grains (wheat, corn, rice, oats, etc.) and its products, fruits, legumes, vegetables, milk, and yogurt. To achieve glycemic control, patients should be advised to monitor their carbohydrate intake. Patients should be instructed to:

- Identify foods containing carbohydrate
- Select healthy carbohydrate choices
- Estimate via carbohydrate counting, exchanges, estimation of portion sizes, plate method and interpreting the nutrition food label, how much carbohydrate is consumed in a meal
- Aim to meet carbohydrate recommendations

Table 13.4 The DASH eating plan at different calorie levels (http://www.dietaryguidelines.gov)

The number of daily servings in a food group vary depending on caloric needs	1,200	1,400	1,600	1,800	2,000	2,600	3,100	Serving sizes
Grains	4–5	5–6	6	6	6–8	10–11	12–13	1 slice bread 1 oz dry cereal ½ cup cooked rice, pasta, or cereal
Vegetables	3–4	3–4	3–4	4–5	4–5	5–6	6	1 cup raw leafy vegetable ½ cup cut-up raw or cooked vegetable ½ cup vegetable juice
Fruits	3–4	4	4	4–5	4–5	5–6	6	1 medium fruit ¼ cup dried fruit ½ cup fresh, frozen, or canned fruit ½ cup fruit juice
Fat-free or low-fat milk and milk products	2–3	2–3	2–3	2–3	2–3	3	3–4	1 cup milk or yogurt 1½ oz cheese
Lean meats, poultry, and fish	3 or less	3–4 or less	3–4 or less	6 or less	6 or less	6 or less	6–9	1 oz cooked meats, poultry, or fish 1 egg
Nuts, seeds, and legumes	3 per week	3 per week	3–4 per week	4 per week	4–5 per week	1	1	⅓ cup or 1½ oz nuts 2 Tbsp peanut butter 2 Tbsp or ½ oz seeds ½ cup cooked legumes (dried beans, peas)
Fats and oils	1	1	2	2–3	2–3	3	4	1 tsp soft margarine 1 tsp vegetable oil 1 Tbsp mayonnaise 1 Tbsp salad dressing
Sweets and added sugars	3 or less per week	3 or less per week	3 or less per week	5 or less per week	5 or less per week	<2	<2	1 Tbsp sugar 1 Tbsp jelly or jam ½ cup sorbet, gelatin dessert 1 cup lemonade
Maximum sodium limited (mg per day)	2,300	2,300	2,300	2,300	2,300	2,300	2,300	

Grains

Encourage patients to choose mostly whole grains. Teach patients to look for the following ingredients on the food label: Brown rice, wild rice, whole-grain sorghum, buckwheat, whole-grain triticale, bulgur (cracked wheat), whole-grain barley, millet, whole-grain corn, popcorn, oatmeal, whole oats/oatmeal, rolled oats, whole rye, quinoa, and whole wheat flour. Advise patients to look for the word "whole" when selecting wheat products to ensure they are selecting whole grain foods — enriched wheat flour is not whole wheat. Grain foods are good sources of carbohydrate. Managing carbohydrate intake is paramount for patients to achieve glycemic control [18].

Fruits and Vegetables

Fruits and vegetables are major sources of folate, magnesium, potassium, dietary fiber, and Vitamins A, C, and K. The 5-A-Day message encourages daily consumption of five servings of fruits and vegetables to reduce risk of coronary heart disease [19]. Among hypertensive individuals, there was a dose–response relationship between fruit and vegetable intake and improvements in endothelial-dependent vasodilation and cardiovascular function providing evidence that even eating one portion a day has potential benefits [20].

Vegetables

Encourage the consumption of a variety of colorful vegetables, especially dark green leafy vegetables and other nonstarchy vegetables such as spinach, kale, collard greens, arugula, Swiss chard, salad greens, broccoli, Brussels sprouts, cauliflower, carrots, tomatoes, among others. Advise patients to fill half of their plates with nonstarchy vegetables. Starchy vegetables, such as potatoes, sweet potatoes, peas, and squash contain more carbohydrate than nonstarchy vegetables and are good sources of potassium. Persons with diabetes should not be discouraged from eating starchy vegetables but should be counseled how to incorporate them into the meal plan.

Fruits

Encourage recommending whole fruit rather than from juice. Fruit may be consumed fresh, frozen, or canned in its own juice or dried. The number of recommended daily servings of fruit should be tailored to the individual's calorie, carbohydrate, and blood glucose targets. Because of their polyphenol content, berries have shown cardio-protective benefits. Raspberries, blueberries, strawberries, peaches, oranges, nectarines, cherries, apples, and pears are lower in glycemic load compared to tropical fruits. The use of glycemic index and load may provide a modest additional benefit over that observed when total carbohydrate is considered alone [21]. In one study, blueberry supplementation showed improved features of metabolic syndrome and related cardiovascular risk factors [22].

Dairy Foods

Encourage fat-free or low-fat milk products. Dairy foods are a major source of dietary calcium. The AI for calcium is 1,000 mg for adults of age 31–50 and 1,200 mg for adults of age 51–70. Examples include fat-free milk or buttermilk; fat-free, low-fat, or reduced-fat cheese; fat-free/low-fat regular or frozen yogurt. Emphasize that whole milk has the same amount of carbohydrate as low-fat and nonfat milk, however the fat content differs. It is important to note that while milk and yogurt contain carbohydrate, cheese does not.

Meats, Poultry, and Fish

Encourage the consumption of lean meats, poultry, and fish. Select only lean; trim away visible fats and skin; broil, roast, or poach and remove fat. Two egg whites have the same protein content as 1 oz meat. Encourage intake of fish high in omega-3 long-chain polyunsaturated fatty acid (LC PUFA) such as salmon, halibut, mackerel, herring, and trout. Reports and studies report diets higher in fish and omega-3 LC-PUFA may reduce cardiovascular risk in diabetes and lower blood pressure [23]. The American Heart Association has recommended the consumption of two weekly servings of fatty fish for all adults without coronary heart disease [24].

Nuts, Seeds, and Legumes

Nuts, seeds, and legumes are rich sources of energy, magnesium, protein, and fiber. Examples include almonds, filberts, mixed nuts, peanuts, walnuts, sunflower seeds, peanut butter, kidney beans, lentils, and split peas. Adding nuts to the diet improves blood lipid profile and reduces the risk of coronary heart disease. Nuts are rich in monounsaturated and polyunsaturated fats. An addition of 60 g of almonds per day has beneficial effects on adiposity, glycemic control, and lipid profile, thus potentially reducing the risk for cardiovascular disease in patients with type 2 diabetes [25]. Individuals with metabolic syndrome showed decreased lipid responsiveness but improved insulin sensitivity after daily intake of just 30 g of mixed nuts (15 g walnuts, 7.5 g almonds, 7.5 g hazelnuts) [26].

Fats and Oils

The DASH study had 27% of calories as fat, including fat in or added to foods. Encourage monounsaturated and polyunsaturated fats and oils such as vegetable oil (canola, corn, olive, safflower, sesame, grapeseed oil) avocadoes as well as the use of soft margarines without partially hydrogenated vegetable oils. The American Diabetes Association [27] dietary fat and cholesterol recommendations in diabetes management include:

- Saturated fat intake should be less than 7% of calories
- Minimize intake of trans fat to lower LDL and increase HDL cholesterol

Olive oil in addition to fruits and vegetables were significantly inversely associated with both systolic and diastolic blood pressures [28]. In a pilot study, use of sesame oil as the sole edible oil had an additive effect in further lowering blood pressure and plasma glucose in hypertensive people with diabetes [29].

Sweets and Added Sugars

Reduce intake of added sugars and avoid sugar sweetened beverages (SSB). They provide extra calories and few essential nutrients. In a study of middle-aged adults, soft drink consumption (one or more 12-oz drink per day) was associated with a higher prevalence and incidence of multiple metabolic risk factors including higher blood pressure [30]. Reducing the consumption of SSB and sugars was significantly associated with reduced blood pressure [31].

Mediterranean Diet and High Blood Pressure Management

The Mediterranean diet has been associated with healthy eating and cardiovascular disease reduction and has conferred improved health outcomes including diabetes [32]. In a meta-analysis of 17 studies, the Mediterranean diet improved fasting glucose and A1C levels for individuals with type 2 diabetes [33]. The Mediterranean diet dietary components are:

- Fruits and vegetables
- Nuts—regular consumption in small quantities
- Legumes
- Olive oil—high in monounsaturated fat and in phenols
- Whole grain cereals/breads
- Wine—regular consumption of low-moderate amounts
- Oily fishes high in omega-3 fatty acids

Table 13.5 Comparison of Mediterranean and DASH eating plans

Eating pattern comparison: Mediterranean, and DASH diet average daily intake at or adjusted to a 2,000 calorie level pattern	Mediterranean patterns, Greece (g), Spain (s)	DASH
Food groups		
Vegetables: total (c)	1.2 (s)—4.1 (g)	2.1
Dark-green (c)	nd	nd
Beans and peas (c)	<0.1 (g)—0.4 (s)	See protein foods
Red and orange (c)	nd	nd
Other (c)	nd	nd
Starchy (c)	nd—0.6 (g)	nd
Fruit and juices (c)	1.4 (s)—2.5 (g) (including nuts)	2.5
Grains: total (oz)	2.0 (s)—5.4 (g)	7.3
Whole grains (oz)	nd	3.9
Milk and milk products (dairy products) (c)	1.0 (g)—2.1 (s)	2.6
Protein foods		
Meat (oz)	3.5 (g)—3.6 (s) (including poultry)	1.4
Poultry (oz)	nd	1.7
Eggs (oz)	nd—1.9 (s)	nd
Fish/seafood (oz)	0.8 (g)—2.4 (s)	1.4
Beans and peas (oz)	See vegetables	0.4 (0.1 c)
Nuts, seeds, and soy products (oz)	See fruits	0.9
Oils (g)	19 (s)—40 (g)	25
Solid fats (g)	nd	nd
Added sugars (g)	nd—24 (g)	12
Alcohol (g)	7.1 (s)—7.9 (g)	nd

Adapted from the eating pattern comparison: usual U.S. intake, Mediterranean, DASH, USDA food patterns, average daily intake or adjusted to a 2,000 calorie level pattern. http://www.dietaryguidelines.gov Accessed August 22, 2011
nd not determined, *c* cups

The Mediterranean diet is limited in:

- Animal protein, especially red meat
- Foods with added sugar
- Eggs—fewer than four per week
- Dairy products

In a study that investigated the individual components of the Mediterranean as a predictor of lower mortality, the dominant components were moderate consumption of ethanol, low consumption of meat and meat products, and high consumption of vegetables, fruits and nuts, olive oil, and legumes [34]. Many components of the DASH and Mediterranean diets are similar and can be integrated (Table 13.5).

Summary

Evidence suggests that emphasis of plant-based foods including vegetables, legumes, nuts, fruits, and sources of monounsaturated and polyunsaturated fats which are also rich in potassium and magnesium and naturally low in sodium is beneficial in the management of hypertension and diabetes. The DASH and Mediterranean diets contain dietary components that have shown to improve glycemic levels and reduce high blood pressure and other metabolic markers. Counseling should emphasize energy balance to maintain or achieve a healthy weight or if not possible, to prevent further weight gain and to reduce sedentary behavior.

References

1. http://www.cdc.gov/diabetes/pubs/factsheet11.htm. Accessed July 21, 2011.
2. Franz MJ, Boucher JL, Green-Pastors J, Powers MAN. Evidenced-based nutrition practice guidelines for diabetes and scope and standards of practice. J Am Diet Assoc. 2008;108 Suppl 1:S52–8.
3. http://www.nhlbi.nih.gov/guidelines/hypertension/jncintro.htm. Accessed July 21, 2011.
4. Forman JP, Stampfer MJ, Curhan GC. Diet and lifestyle risk factors associated with incident hypertension in women. J Am Med Assoc. 2009;302:401–11.
5. Neter JE, Stam BE, Kok FJ, Grobbee DE, Geleijnse JM. Influence of weight reduction on blood pressure. A meta-analysis of randomized controlled trials. Hypertension. 2003;42: 878–84.
6. He J, Whelton PK, Appel LJ, Charleston J, Klag MJ. Long-term effects of weight loss and dietary sodium reduction on incidence of hypertension. Hypertension. 2000;35:544–9.
7. Dietary Guidelines for Americans 2010. http://www.dietaryguidelines.gov. Accessed August 12, 2011.
8. U.S. Department of Health and Human Services. 2008 Physical Activity Guidelines for Americans. Washington (DC): U.S. Department of Health and Human Services; 2008. Office of Disease Prevention and Health Promotion Publication No. U0036. http://www.health.gov/paguidelines. Accessed August 12, 2011.
9. http://www.nhlbi.nih.gov/health/health-topics/topics/dash. Accessed July 21, 2011.
10. Blumenthal JA, et al. Effects of the DASH diet alone and in combination with exercise and weight loss on blood pressure and cardiovascular biomarkers in men and women with high blood pressure. Arch Intern Med. 2010;170(2):126–35.
11. Dietary Guidelines for Americans http://www.cnpp.usda.gov/dgas2010-dgacreport.htm and http://www.dietaryguidelines.gov. Accessed July 27, 2011
12. Houston MC. The importance of potassium in managing hypertension. Curr Hypertens Rep. 2011;13(4):309–17.
13. http://www.ars.usda.gov/SP2UserFiles/Place/12354500/Data/SR22/ nutrlist/sr22w306.pdf. Accessed July 27, 2011.
14. Yamori Y, Mizushima S. A review of the link between dietary magnesium and cardiovascular risk. J Cardiovasc Risk. 2000;7:31–5.
15. Mizushima S, Cappuccio FP, Nichols R, Elliott P. Dietary magnesium intake and blood pressure: a qualitative overview of the observational studies. J Hum Hypertens. 1998;12:447–53.
16. Song Y, Sesso HD, Manson JE, Cook NR, Buring JE, Liu S. Dietary magnesium intake and risk of incident hypertension among middle-aged and older US women in a 10-year follow-up study. Am J Cardiol. 2006;98:1616–21.

17. Sarkkinen ES, Kastarinen MJ, Niskanen TH, Karjalainen PH, Venäläinen TM, Udani JK, et al. Feasibility and antihypertensive effect of replacing regular salt with mineral salt -rich in magnesium and potassium- in subjects with mildly elevated blood pressure. Nutr J. 2011;10:88.
18. Franz MJ, Powers MA, Leontos C, Holzmeister LA, Kulkarni K, Monk A, et al. The evidence for medical nutrition therapy for type 1 and type 2 diabetes in adults. J Am Diet Assoc. 2010;110:1852–89.
19. http://www.fruitsandveggiesmatter.gov/index.html. Accessed July 29, 2011.
20. McCall DO, McGartland CP, McKinley MC, Patterson CC, Sharpe P, McCance DR, et al. Dietary intake of fruits and vegetables improves microvascular function in hypertensive subjects in a dose-dependent manner. Circulation. 2009;119(16):2153–60.
21. American Diabetes Association. Nutrition recommendations and interventions for diabetes: a position statement of the American Diabetes Association. Diabetes Care. 2008;31:S61–78.
22. Basu A, Du M, Leyva MJ, Sanchez K, Betts NM, Wu M, et al. Blueberries decrease cardiovascular risk factors in obese men and women with metabolic syndrome. J Nutr. 2010;140(9): 1582–7.
23. McEwen B, Morel-Kopp MC, Tofler G, Ward C. Effect of omega-3 fish oil on cardiovascular risk in diabetes. Diabetes Educ. 2010;36:565–84.
24. Kris-Etherton PM, Harris WS, Appel LJ. Fish consumption, fish oil, omega-3 fatty acids, and cardiovascular disease. Circulation. 2002;106:2747–57.
25. Li SC, Liu YH, Liu JF, Chang WH, Chen CM, Chen CY. Almond consumption improved glycemic control and lipid profiles in patients with Type 2 diabetes. Metabolism. 2011;60(4): 474–4479.
26. Casas-Agustench P, Lopez-Uriarte P, Bulló M, Ross E, Cabré-Vila JJ, Salas-Salvado J. Effects of one serving of mixed nuts on serum lipids, insulin resistance, and inflammatory markers in patients with the metabolic syndrome. Nutr Metab Cardiovasc Dis. 2011;21(2):126–35.
27. American Diabetes Association. Standards of medical care in diabetes. Diabetes Care. 2010;33:S23–5.
28. Psaltopoulou T, Naska A, Orfanos P, Trichopoulos D, Mountokalakis T, Trichopoulou A. Olive oil, the Mediterranean diet, and arterial blood pressure: the Greek European Prospective Investigation into Cancer and Nutrition (EPIC) study. Am J Clin Nutr. 2004;80:1012–8.
29. Sankar D, Rao MR, Sambandam G, Pugalendi KV. A pilot study of open label sesame oil in hypertensive diabetics. J Med Food. 2006;9(3):408–12.
30. Dhinga R, Sullivan L, Jacques P, Wang TJ, Fox CS, Meigs JB, et al. Soft drink consumption and risk of developing cardiometabolic risk factors and the metabolic syndrome in middle-aged adults in the community. Circulation. 2007;116:480–8.
31. Chen L, Caballero B, Mitchell DC, Loria C, Lin PH, Champagne C, et al. Reducing consumption of sugar-sweetened beverages is associated with reduced blood pressure. A prospective study among United States adults. Circulation. 2010;121:2398–406.
32. Martínez-González MA, de la Fuente-Arrillaga C, Nunez-Cordoba JM, Basterra-Gortari FJ, Beunza JJ, Vazquez Z, et al. Adherence to Mediterranean diet and risk of developing diabetes: prospective cohort study. Br Med J. 2008;336:1348–51.
33. Esposito K, Maiorino MI, Ceriello A, Giugliano D. Prevention and control of type 2 diabetes by mediterranean diet: a systematic review. Diabetes Res Clin Pract. 2010;89:97–102.
34. Trichopoulou A, Bamia C, Trichopoulos D. Anatomy of health effects of Mediterranean diet: Greek EPIC prospective cohort study. Br Med J. 2009;338:b2337.

Chapter 14
Novel Pharmacological Approaches in Hypertension Treatment

Edgar Lerma and George L. Bakris

Treatment of hypertension remains a challenging task despite the tremendous breakthroughs and advancements in the field. Hypertension is defined as systolic blood pressure (SBP) above 140 mmHg and diastolic blood pressure (DBP) above 90 mmHg. The Seventh Report of the Joint National Committee on Prevention, Detection, Evaluation, and Treatment of High Blood Pressure currently recommends treatment to be initiated with the goal of lowering below the target of 140/90 mmHg. This guideline goal reduces cardiovascular morbidity and mortality.

Following lifestyle modifications, antihypertensive therapy is recommended based on compelling indication. Use of angiotensin-converting enzyme inhibitor (ACEI), angiotensin receptor blocker (ARB), diuretics, beta blocker (BB), or calcium channel blocker (CCB) is warranted as initial agents. If the blood pressure goals are more than 20 mmHg above goal for systolic and above 10 mmHg above goal for diastolic pressure, initiation of two agents has been suggested. Most important adjunctive measures include regular physical activity, weight loss if overweight/obese, diet rich in fruits and vegetables, as well as decreased daily sodium intake [1]. Analysis of the National Health and Nutrition Survey 2006–2008 manifested a rise in individuals diagnosed with hypertension; however, it reported the highest ever control rates, i.e., >50% [2]. However, the remaining problem is the lack of blood pressure control estimated to be almost 41% in all groups. With an estimated 1.5 billion people worldwide with a diagnosis of hypertension by 2025, the proportion of patients with the potential for serious health problems related to uncontrolled hypertension is only enlarging [3]. The failure to attain recommended blood pressure goals in the treatment of hypertension is attributed to either (a) true resistant hypertension

E. Lerma
Section of Nephrology, University of Illinois at Chicago School of Medicine, Chicago, IL, USA

G.L. Bakris, M.D. (✉)
Department of Medicine, ASH Comprehensive Hypertension Center, University of Chicago Medical Center, 5841 S. Maryland Avenue, MC1027, Chicago, IL 60637, USA
e-mail: gbakris@gmail.com

S.I. McFarlane and G.L. Bakris (eds.), *Diabetes and Hypertension: Evaluation and Management*, Contemporary Diabetes, DOI 10.1007/978-1-60327-357-2_14,
© Springer Science+Business Media New York 2012

or (b) uncontrolled hypertension that includes under treatment, inadequate evaluation for secondary causes of hypertension, or non-adherence to medication regimens.

True resistant hypertension is defined as a lack of achieving blood pressure goals when therapy is maximized using at least three maximally tolerated doses of antihypertensive agents, one of which is a diuretic [4]. Novel therapies may improve control rates but ultimately appropriate dosing of these medications, enhanced tolerability, and improvement of adherence to medication regimens are necessary for control rates to improve.

The major advances in hypertension therapy discussed in this chapter focus on (a) new uses for established monotherapies in various combinations, (b) fixed-dose combinations and cardiovascular outcomes, (c) novel uses of fixed-dose combinations as initial therapy, (d) use of vaccines, (e) compounds that are in Phase 1 testing, (f) carotid baroreceptor stimulation, and (g) renal nerve ablation.

New Uses for Monotherapies in Combination

Mineralocorticoid Antagonists

Mineralocorticoid antagonists are well known to augment favorable outcomes in hypertensive patients with advanced heart failure and CAD [5]. Addition of aldosterone blockade to ARB or ACEI plus thiazide diuretic has significantly improved blood pressure control in individuals with resistant hypertension who do not have primary aldosteronism. In some studies, an average decrease of 26 mmHg in SBP and 11 mmHg in DBP at 6 months is noted when compared to controls [6]. Data from the Anglo-Scandinavian Cardiac Outcomes Trial (ASCOT)—Blood Pressure Lowering Arm demonstrate that addition of spironolactone as a fourth agent to the patients with resistant hypertension augments decreases in SBP for 21.9 mmHg and DBP for 9.5 mmHg [7]. Apart from heart failure, however, the cardiovascular outcomes remain largely unstudied for medication regimens that have aldosterone blockade as part of "the cocktail." In addition, the concern regarding side effects, namely, hyperkalemia and increases in serum creatinine, remains, although they are restricted for the most part to patients with an estimated glomerular filtration rate below 45 mL/min and serum potassium above 4.5 mEq/L when therapy is started [8].

Renin Inhibitors

While renin was a target investigated in the 1980s, the first antihypertensive agent emerged at the dawn of the twenty-first century. Currently, the only approved renin inhibitor in the United States is aliskiren. The data presented are consistent with excellent side-effect profile, not much different when compared to placebo.

Evaluation of effectiveness as compared to placebo has shown excellent results in several trials [9]. The efficacy was assessed in patients with mild to moderate hypertension (DBP >95 and >110 mmHg), without comorbidities including diabetes, CAD, and stroke. The comparison was made with placebo and across different dose regimens and with ARB. Combination treatment with aliskiren and ramipril has achieved better BP than in either of them alone [10]. The ultimate test of when aliskiren will provide a meaningful impact on mortality reduction will be known in 2012, when the ALTITUDE trial is completed. This trial evaluates cardiovascular and renal outcomes in more than 10,000 patients [11].

Endothelin Receptor Antagonists

Nonselective endothelin receptor antagonists have been around for more than 20 years; however, their efficacy as antihypertensive agents is questioned. More recently, data on the efficacy of selective endothelin A receptor inhibitors have presented promising results. The selective type A endothelin receptor blocker, darusentan, was evaluated as an additive therapy to the hypertensive patient groups that were diagnosed with resistant hypertensions and already on a recommended regimen as defined above compared to the addition of placebo. A primary endpoint of systolic blood pressure improvement toward goal has been noted with all three different dosings of darusentan as compared to placebo. In this trial, 23% of patients in the placebo group achieved goal blood pressure (<140/90 mmHg of <130/80 mmHg for renal impairment and diabetes) compared to 41–53% over darusentan group [12]. A recently completed secondary study using 24 h ambulatory monitoring also demonstrated darusentan to be superior over active therapy and placebo, although the primary endpoint of office blood pressure at a single time point failed to meet the endpoint and, thus, the trial was viewed as not successful [13]. The safety profile of this class is questionable, however, as worsening peripheral edema and hemodilution have been reported as common occurrences.

Fixed-Dose Combination Therapy

Most of the current approaches to antihypertensive treatment advocate use of monotherapy even though the combination strategy is advocated in patients who have initial BP readings higher than 20/10 mmHg above the goal of <140/90 mmHg.

Early studies clearly demonstrated that initial therapy with a fixed-dose combination was able to achieve the recommended blood pressure goal in patients with type 2 diabetes faster than conventional monotherapy [14]. At 3 months, more participants in the combination group achieved treatment goal (63% combination vs. 37% conventional; $p=0.002$). Moreover, blood pressure control rates between the fixed-dose combination group (without HCTZ) to the conventional group (receiving

HCTZ) after 3 months showed an even greater disparity in blood pressure goal achievement (87% combination without HCTZ vs. 37% conventional group with HCTZ; $p=0.0001$). This study paved the way for a fixed-dose combination approach for achieving blood pressure goal in that it was safe and more efficacious than the conventional methods. Additionally, the combination dual therapy would be an attractive option for several reasons including improving adherence, avoiding frequent visits for dose adjustments, offsetting individual medication side effects, and complimentary hemodynamic benefits if medication classes are chosen appropriately with regard to their modes of action [15, 16].

Data from the first trial to randomize two different fixed-dose combinations, ACCOMPLISH, studied a patient population with high cardiovascular risk and a mean age of 69 years. The authors' demonstrated superiority of a calcium channel blocker (CCB)/angiotensin-converting enzyme inhibitor (ACEI) combination over a thiazide diuretic/ACEI combination therapy for reducing the primary endpoint is defined as a composite of cardiovascular events and death from any cause [17]. Both patient groups in this trial had similar baseline characteristics and reached similar blood pressure targets of 131/73 and 132/74 mmHg after an average 30-month follow-up. Moreover, the lack of difference in blood pressure between groups was confirmed by 24 h ambulatory monitoring [18].

At present, there are seven classes of antihypertensive agents, with multiple members under each class. These are all summarized and recommendations are made in the recent position paper by the American Society of Hypertension (ASH) [16]. Since the focus of this chapter is to discuss novel agents, the reader is referred to the ASH position paper [16] for full details.

Triple Combination

ARB + CCB + Diuretic

Recently, reports from a phase 3, randomized, parallel-group multicenter study (TRINITY) of triple versus dual combination, fixed-dose antihypertensive therapy in patients with moderate to severe hypertension showed superiority of the former [19, 20]. In both cases, addition of the thiazide diuretic to the dual combination of amlodipine and an angiotensin receptor blocker led to further enhanced BP reduction.

Vaccines

Angiotensin I and angiotensin II have been targets of vaccines against hypertension that are currently under development. Despite several studies demonstrating comparable BP reduction and efficacy versus classical pharmacological agents, the challenges involving the development of such vaccines pertain to not only the quality, but also the quantity of induced antibodies. Similarly, small sample sizes remain a significant limitation of the above studies.

PMD3117

Phase I and II testing of the angiotensin I vaccine PMD3117 attested to its safety and immunogenicity in humans. However, its lack of efficacy in reducing BP has been attributed to the insufficient quantity of induced antibodies [21].

CYT006-AngQb

CYT006-AngQb is a virus-shaped noninfectious particle that is coupled with angiotensin II, a known vasoconstrictor. Such coupling induces the formation of antibodies against angiotensin II, thereby potentially reducing its effects on vasoconstriction. As compared to placebo, CYT006-AngQb was shown to reduce ambulatory BP. It was particularly effective in reducing early morning (during which time, most cardiovascular events occur) SBP and DBP by 25 and 13 mmHg, respectively [22].

At present, CYT006-AngQb is the only effective vaccine tested in humans that has been shown to effectively reduce BP (−9/−4 mmHg). With a relatively long half-life of 4 months, it has also been suggested that the affinity (rather than the titers) of the antibodies is the major factor that determines its effectiveness.

ATR12181

ATR12181 is a vaccine against the AngII-type Ia receptor and has been shown to reduce BP by 17 mmHg in spontaneous hypertensive rats (SHRs) [23]. These data on vaccines, taken together, suggest that reduction in blood pressure can be achieved by inducing immunity against targets in the RAAS. The target antigen and selection of adjuvant are crucial factors determining the effectiveness and safety of the vaccine. While CYT006-AngQb (angiotensin II vaccine) reduces blood pressure in humans, the results were not reproducible with more frequent dosing. Vaccines for hypertension are still in the early phase.

Novel Targets

More than 20 new compounds are under investigation as possible new antihypertensive agents. These include aldosterone synthetase inhibitors, adenosine 1 receptor antagonists, AMP activated protein kinase (AMK), acetyl Co-enzyme A carboxylase, and many others. Some of these are in Phase 2 trials such as the aldosterone synthase inhibitors. Others have been studied such as adenosine 1 receptor antagonists and while efficacious have side-effect profiles that mitigate against their continued development.

It is clear that since hypertension is a polygenic disorder, it will require combinations of multi-target therapy to fully control [24]. The ideal combination remains to be determined and even that will vary depending on the genotype and phenotype of a given patient. New agents targeting specific cellular mechanisms will aid in developing such combinations.

Novel Nondrug Approaches to Control Hypertension

The sympathetic nervous system plays one of the most important roles in the pathophysiology of essential hypertension. Pharmacologic resources employed in controlling of this mechanism have not so far been very potent in regulating blood pressure. Recently, more focus has been given to techniques that mechanically interfere with the sympathetic outflow in these individuals. The two include catheter-based renal sympathetic denervation and carotid sinus stimulator.

Renal Nerve Ablation

The kidney contributes to the development and maintenance of elevated blood pressure in many different ways, one being efferent and afferent sympathetic system, which is located near the renal arteries walls. This renal nerve stimulation has been implicated in contributing to the maintenance of hypertension through increased sympathetic nervous system activity in the kidney [25]. Specifically, this increased nerve activity is postulated to increase renal vascular resistance subsequently initiating a cascade of events that include overactivation of RAS and increased fluid and salt retention [25]. A pilot study in hypertensive patients by Krum et al. [26] has assessed safety and efficacy of percutaneous, catheter-based removal of sympathetic renal nerves in humans after several investigational and successful attempts in animals. The procedure is performed percutaneously with a catheter connected to the radiofrequency generator. This study had 50 individuals with resistant hypertension defined as those with a SBP > 160 mmHg while receiving three or more antihypertensive agents, one of which was a diuretic. Denervation was bilateral and blood pressure response was monitored at 3, 6, 9, and 12 months post-procedure with significant average reductions of 14/10, 21/10, 22/11, 24/11, and 27/17 mmHg, respectively, in 45 individuals. There were 13% non-responders in the group. The safety profile, which was the primary endpoint, was promising as only one patient suffered a renal artery dissection and another had a pseudoaneurysm of the femoral site both with favorable outcomes. There were no severe adverse events noted 6 months after the procedure including deterioration of renal function. One benefit of the procedure was restoration of blood pressure dipping pattern.

In addition to the aforementioned direct effects of the procedure, it is also important to note that renal denervation decreased renin secretion by about 50% [26, 27]. This may potentially influence central sympathetic outflow by altering circulating angiotensin II levels. Other effects of renal denervation included improved cardiac baroreflex sensitivity (from 7.8 to 11.7 ms/mmHg), and a significant reduction of LV mass compared to baseline (from 184 to 169 g; 78.8 to 73.1 g/m^2), as demonstrated by cardiac MRI, after 12 months of follow-up [26, 27].

This approach certainly looks promising; however, it does need large-scale studies to assess its long-term usefulness and potential side effects.

Rheos

Baroreceptor triggering is one of the physiologic mechanisms involved in a blood pressure control. It is activated by vascular distension secondary to the rise in systemic blood pressure and consecutive propagation of impulses to the medulla activating parasympathetic nuclei and inhibiting sympathetic outflow [28]. This mechanism has been a target of blood pressure control for a long time with good results in animal studies, but only gaining substantial attention; recently this translated into the studies involving human subjects. The current approach involves a carotid sinus stimulator marketed as Rheos. This device is implanted bilaterally around both carotid sinuses. An artificial pulse generator implanted subcutaneously provides a predetermined electrical impulse to stimulate the carotid sinus to elicit a tonic neuronal response [28]. Thus far, several small studies in United States and Europe have assessed procedure safety and tolerability. The effects on blood pressure in humans are described in a small study by Illig et al. [29] who evaluated ten individuals, all diagnosed with resistant hypertension, using the aforementioned definition. These individuals were on average of six antihypertensive medications with a mean blood pressure prior to enrollment of 175/101 mmHg. The estimated postoperative drop in blood pressure was 41 mmHg for SBP and 19 mmHg for DBP with a device peak response at average of 4.8 V [30].

Similarly, European investigators found a significant blood pressure improvement in hypertensive individuals diagnosed with resistant hypertension. Heusser et al. [31] showed that electrical field stimulation of the carotid baroreceptors acutely reduced sympathetic nerve activity in a subgroup of patients with refractory hypertension, resulting in decreased plasma renin concentration and BP. Interestingly, despite continued stimulation throughout the cardiac cycle, no symptoms indicative of baroreflex dysfunction were reported. The authors suggested that the maintenance of lower BP readings results from baroreceptor regulation of heart rate, and muscle sympathetic nerve activity was most likely due to a leftward shift of the baroreflex curves and their operating points.

The initial mean maximal changes in systolic blood pressure were 28 mmHg and in diastolic blood pressure 16 mmHg that was sustained in a follow-up of 4 months. The results seem promising and initially assessed safety profiles are mostly related to procedure-related infections and hypoglossal nerve injury, which improved in a follow-up [32]. A study looking into the structural integrity after implantation of the carotid sinus stimulator showed no evidence of development of carotid stenosis or injury [30]. The Device Based Therapy in Hypertension Trial (DEBuT-HT), a multicenter, prospective, non-randomized feasibility trial started in Europe in March 2004, seeks to demonstrate the safety and efficacy of the Rheos Baroreflex Hypertension Therapy System in patients with refractory hypertension despite full pharmacologic therapy, and is still ongoing [33].

Large-scale studies are under way and an answer to the feasibility of this device will be apparent within the next couple of years. Similarly, research should also focus on developing a more portable (smaller size and weight) device with a longer longevity (battery). Newer methodology has resulted in improved and much longer battery life. Additionally, newer technology allows for unilateral placement of the device.

Glossary

ACCOMPLISH Avoiding cardiovascular events through combination therapy in patients living with systolic hypertension.

ALTITUDE Aliskiren trial in type 2 diabetes using cardio-renal endpoints.

ASCOT Anglo-Scandinavian cardiac outcomes trial.

ASH American Society of Hypertension.

ATR12181 Vaccine against the angiotensin II-type Ia receptor.

CAD Coronary artery disease.

CYT006 AngQb is a virus-shaped noninfectious particle that is coupled with angiotensin II, a known vasoconstrictor.

LV Left ventricle.

MRI Magnetic resonance imaging.

Novel therapy An approach to reduce blood pressure that has either not been approved yet or recently approved and has less than 5 years of clinical experience.

PMD3117 A vaccine against angiotensin I.

RAS Renal artery stenosis.

Renin inhibitors Inhibit the rate limiting enzyme (renin) for the genesis or angiotensin II.

Resistant hypertension Lack of achieving blood pressure goal (<140/90 mmHg) using at least three maximally tolerated doses of antihypertensive agents one of which is a diuretic.

TRINITY Multicenter, randomized, double-blind, parallel-group study of triple combination treatment with olmesartan, amlodipine, and hydrochlorothiazide compared with dual combinations of the individual components.

References

1. Chobanian AV, Bakris GL, Black HR, Cushman WC, Green LA, Izzo Jr JL, et al. Seventh report of the Joint National Committee on Prevention, Detection, Evaluation, and Treatment of High Blood Pressure. Hypertension. 2003;42(6):1206–52.
2. Egan BM, Zhao Y, Axon RN. US trends in prevalence, awareness, treatment, and control of hypertension, 1988–2008. J Am Med Assoc. 2010;303(20):2043–50.
3. Kearney PM, Whelton M, Reynolds K, Muntner P, Whelton PK, He J. Global burden of hypertension: analysis of worldwide data. Lancet. 2005;365(9455):217–23.
4. Sarafidis PA, Bakris GL. Resistant hypertension: an overview of evaluation and treatment. J Am Coll Cardiol. 2008;52(22):1749–57.
5. Verma A, Solomon SD. Optimizing care of heart failure after acute MI with an aldosterone receptor antagonist. Curr Heart Fail Rep. 2007;4(4):183–9.
6. Nishizaka MK, Zaman MA, Calhoun DA. Efficacy of low-dose spironolactone in subjects with resistant hypertension. Am J Hypertens. 2003;16(11 Pt 1):925–30.
7. Chapman N, Dobson J, Wilson S, Dahlof B, Sever PS, Wedel H, et al. Effect of spironolactone on blood pressure in subjects with resistant hypertension. Hypertension. 2007;49(4):839–45.
8. Khosla N, Kalaitzidis R, Bakris GL. Predictors of hyperkalemia risk following hypertension control with aldosterone blockade. Am J Nephrol. 2009;30(5):418–24.
9. Musini VM, Fortin PM, Bassett K, Wright JM. Blood pressure lowering efficacy of renin inhibitors for primary hypertension: a Cochrane systematic review. J Hum Hypertens. 2009;23(8):495–502.
10. Uresin Y, Taylor AA, Kilo C, Tschope D, Santonastaso M, Ibram G, et al. Efficacy and safety of the direct renin inhibitor aliskiren and ramipril alone or in combination in patients with diabetes and hypertension. J Renin Angiotensin Aldosterone Syst. 2007;8(4):190–8.
11. Parving HH, Brenner BM, McMurray JJ, de ZD, Haffner SM, Solomon SD, et al. Aliskiren trial in type 2 diabetes using cardio-renal endpoints (ALTITUDE): rationale and study design. Nephrol Dial Transplant. 2009;24(5):1663–71.
12. Weber MA, Black H, Bakris G, Krum H, Linas S, Weiss R, et al. A selective endothelin-receptor antagonist to reduce blood pressure in patients with treatment-resistant hypertension: a randomised, double-blind, placebo-controlled trial. Lancet. 2009;374(9699):1423–31.
13. Bakris GL, Lindholm LH, Black HR, Krum H, Linas S, Linseman JV, et al. Divergent results using clinic and ambulatory blood pressures. Report of a darusentan-resistant hypertension trial. Hypertension. 2010;56(5):824–30.
14. Bakris GL, Weir MR. Achieving goal blood pressure in patients with type 2 diabetes: conventional versus fixed-dose combination approaches. J Clin Hypertens (Greenwich). 2003;5(3):202–9.
15. Mancia G, Failla M, Grappiolo A, Giannattasio C. Present and future role of combination treatment in hypertension. J Cardiovasc Pharmacol. 1998;31 Suppl 2:S41–4.
16. Gradman AH, Basile JN, Carter BL, Bakris GL, Materson BJ, Black HR, et al. Combination therapy in hypertension. J Am Soc Hypertens. 2010;4(2):90–8.
17. Jamerson K, Weber MA, Bakris GL, Dahlof B, Pitt B, Shi V, et al. Benazepril plus amlodipine or hydrochlorothiazide for hypertension in high-risk patients. N Engl J Med. 2008;359(23):2417–28.
18. Jamerson KA, Bakris GL, Weber MA. 24-Hour ambulatory blood pressure in the ACCOMPLISH trial. N Engl J Med. 2010;363(1):98.
19. Oparil S, Melino M, Lee J, Fernandez V, Heyrman R. Triple therapy with olmesartan medoxomil, amlodipine besylate, and hydrochlorothiazide in adult patients with hypertension: The TRINITY multicenter, randomized, double-blind, 12-week, parallel-group study. Clin Ther. 2010;32(7):1252–69.
20. Calhoun DA, Crikelair NA, Yen J, Glazer RD. Amlodipine/valsartan/hydrochlorothiazide triple combination therapy in moderate/severe hypertension: secondary analyses evaluating efficacy and safety. Adv Ther. 2009;26(11):1012–23.

21. Brown MJ, Coltart J, Gunewardena K, Ritter JM, Auton TR, Glover JF. Randomized double-blind placebo-controlled study of an angiotensin immunotherapeutic vaccine (PMD3117) in hypertensive subjects. Clin Sci (Lond). 2004;107(2):167–73.

22. Tissot AC, Maurer P, Nussberger J, Sabat R, Pfister T, Ignatenko S, et al. Effect of immunisation against angiotensin II with CYT006-AngQb on ambulatory blood pressure: a double-blind, randomised, placebo-controlled phase IIa study. Lancet. 2008;371(9615):821–7.

23. Ambuhl PM, Tissot AC, Fulurija A, Maurer P, Nussberger J, Sabat R, et al. A vaccine for hypertension based on virus-like particles: preclinical efficacy and phase I safety and immunogenicity. J Hypertens. 2007;25(1):63–72.

24. Rafiq S, Anand S, Roberts R. Genome-wide association studies of hypertension: have they been fruitful? J Cardiovasc Transl Res. 2010;3(3):189–96.

25. Katholi RE, Rocha-Singh KJ, Goswami NJ, Sobotka PA. Renal nerves in the maintenance of hypertension: a potential therapeutic target. Curr Hypertens Rep. 2010;12(3):196–204.

26. Krum H, Schlaich M, Whitbourn R, Sobotka PA, Sadowski J, Bartus K, et al. Catheter-based renal sympathetic denervation for resistant hypertension: a multicentre safety and proof-of-principle cohort study. Lancet. 2009;373(9671):1275–81.

27. Schlaich MP, Sobotka PA, Krum H, Lambert E, Esler MD. Renal sympathetic-nerve ablation for uncontrolled hypertension. N Engl J Med. 2009;361(9):932–4.

28. Filippone JD, Bisognano JD. Baroreflex stimulation in the treatment of hypertension. Curr Opin Nephrol Hypertens. 2007;16(5):403–8.

29. Illig KA, Levy M, Sanchez L, Trachiotis GD, Shanley C, Irwin E, et al. An implantable carotid sinus stimulator for drug-resistant hypertension: surgical technique and short-term outcome from the multicenter phase II Rheos feasibility trial. J Vasc Surg. 2006;44(6):1213–8.

30. Sanchez LA, Illig K, Levy M, Jaff M, Trachiotis G, Shanley C, et al. Implantable carotid sinus stimulator for the treatment of resistant hypertension: local effects on carotid artery morphology. Ann Vasc Surg. 2010;24(2):178–84.

31. Heusser K, Tank J, Engeli S, Diedrich A, Menne J, Eckert S, et al. Carotid baroreceptor stimulation, sympathetic activity, baroreflex function, and blood pressure in hypertensive patients. Hypertension. 2010;55(3):619–26.

32. Tordoir JH, Scheffers I, Schmidli J, Savolainen H, Liebeskind U, Hansky B, et al. An implantable carotid sinus baroreflex activating system: surgical technique and short-term outcome from a multi-center feasibility trial for the treatment of resistant hypertension. Eur J Vasc Endovasc Surg. 2007;33(4):414–21.

33. Scheffers IJ, Kroon AA, Tordoir JH, de Leeuw PW. Rheos baroreflex hypertension therapy system to treat resistant hypertension. Expert Rev Med Devices. 2008;5(1):33–9.

Index

S.I. McFarlane and G.L. Bakris (eds.), *Diabetes and Hypertension: Evaluation
and Management*, Contemporary Diabetes, DOI 10.1007/978-1-60327-357-2,
© Springer Science+Business Media New York 2012